Handbook of Dermato

For Philippa

Handbook of Dermatology

D.J. Barker MA MB MRCP
Consultant Dermatologist, Bradford Royal Infirmary,
Duckworth Lane, Bradford

OXFORD

BLACKWELL SCIENTIFIC PUBLICATIONS

LONDON EDINBURGH BOSTON

MELBOURNE PARIS BERLIN VIENNA

© 1990 by
Blackwell Scientific Publications
Editorial Offices:
Osney Mead, Oxford OX2 0EL
25 John Street, London WC1N 2BL
23 Ainslie Place, Edinburgh EH3 6AJ
3 Cambridge Center, Cambridge,
  Massachusetts 02142, USA
54 University Street, Carlton
  Victoria 3053, Australia

First published 1990

Set by Setrite Typesetters, Hong Kong
Printed and bound in Great Britain at
The Alden Press, Oxford

DISTRIBUTORS

Marston Book Services Ltd
PO Box 87
Oxford OX2 0DT
(*Orders*: Tel. 0865 791155
       Fax: 0865 791927
       Telex: 837515)

USA
  Mosby–Year Book, Inc.
  200 North LaSalle Street
  Chicago, Illinois 60601
  (*Orders*: Tel: (312) 726–9733)

Canada
  Mosby–Year Book, Inc.
  5240 Finch Avenue East
  Scarborough, Ontario
  (*Orders*: Tel: (416) 298–1588)

Australia
  Blackwell Scientific
  Publications
  (Australia) Pty Ltd
  54 University Street
  Carlton, Victoria 3053
  (*Orders*: Tel: (03) 347–0300)

British Library
Cataloguing in Publication Data

Barker, D.J.
  Handbook of dermatology.
  1. Medicine. Dermatology
  I. Title
  616.5

ISBN 0–632–02444–5

Contents

Appendices

Colour plates appear between pp. 88 and 89

Preface

While writing this book I have tried to keep in mind the needs of general practitioners, vocational trainees, medical students, dermatology nurses and pharmacists rather than hospital specialists. All these groups need an up-to-date guide to the agents used to treat common skin disease, and a succinct account of the diseases themselves.

Lengthy discussion and references to the literature seem inappropriate in an introductory textbook. As a result what follows may appear excessively dogmatic and didactic. I hope this will be forgiven if it is also safe and sensible. To increase the practical value of the book some specimen patient advice sheets together with a bibliography are collected in an appendix. As far as possible I have made the drugs and preparations mentioned consistent with the British National Formulary (BNF) of March 1990. The composition of the very few exceptions to this rule will be found in a separate formulary. British readers must remember that some drugs described, such as topical minoxidil, are not usually prescribable within the National Health Service. Others, like etretinate, are available for hospital use only.

I hope to convince readers that the successful management of patients with skin disorders does not require the instant and infallible recognition of rare diseases and syndromes, but rather a thorough knowledge of the common conditions with a logical strategy for diagnosis and treatment. Finally it should be remembered that skin disorders vary in presentation and incidence among different ethnic groups.

D.J.B.

Acknowledgements

I must acknowledge my debt to Dr L.G. Millard who first suggested that I should write this book, and to Dr W. J. Cunliffe who has encouraged my medical writing for many years. Dr J.M. Foy read the first draft of the manuscript and made many helpful suggestions. Any errors and omissions that remain despite these interventions are entirely my responsibility.

1: Principles of diagnosis

Before examining a patient with a skin disorder it is helpful to take a preliminary history which establishes mutual rapport and enables the diagnostic possibilities to be substantially reduced. Establish when the problem began, what sites were involved and how it has subsequently progressed. The presence or absence of pruritus is very helpful in reaching a diagnosis (Table 1.1).

Table 1.1 Intensely itchy skin disorders

Scabies
Insect bites
Atopic eczema
Urticaria
Lichen planus
Dermatitis herpetiformis

It is wise to enquire if any other family members have a skin disease, or asthma and hay fever. Many patients with psoriasis, atopic eczema, neurofibromatosis, or indeed scabies, will be aware of affected relatives.

Rashes are one of the most common adverse effects of drugs and drug eruptions have replaced syphilis as 'the great mimic'. Ask about any previous treatment applied to the rash. A topical steroid can temporarily suppress, but not of course eradicate, a fungal infection. When referring a patient to a dermatologist try to provide a full drug history. Apart from all other considerations it is frustrating to make therapeutic suggestions only to have them greeted by the patient with 'my own doctor tried that; it didn't work!'

For all except the most trivial problems a general inspection of the skin is necessary. Patients do not always anticipate the need for this and should receive a full explanation before being asked to undress. Muslim women may well have religious objections to examination by a man.

1

When you examine the skin observe the morphology of single lesions and also the way in which the lesions are distributed over the body. Individually the umbilicated papules of molluscum contagiosum or the burrows of scabies should be diagnostic. An inflammatory rash in a dermatomal distribution is likely to be shingles. Scaly erythematous plaques on the low back, elbows and knees would of course be characteristic of psoriasis. The lesions of some spontaneously occurring disorders will localize in sites of trauma. This is termed the Köbner phenomenon (Table 1.2).

Table 1.2 Skin disease associated with the Köbner phenomenon

Psoriasis
Lichen planus
Molluscum contagiosum
Vitiligo

Changes such as vesiculation, scaling and hypopigmentation are epidermal in origin. Erythema is a dermal change. Changes in both cutaneous layers can result in skin thickening.

Try not to be a merely passive observer but actively search for confirmatory physical signs. Psoriasis often produces well demarcated scaly scalp patches, nail pitting and onycholysis. Lichen planus and erythema multiforme frequently involve the mouth. Erythematous penile nodules are a virtually diagnostic feature of scabies.

After examining a patient you will wish to ask supplemental questions. The existence of hand eczema should certainly suggest the need for an occupational history. Scalp ringworm or papular urticaria would naturally lead to enquiries about domestic pets. Enquire if there has been recent foreign travel. Over the last few years in Northern England I have seen patients with leprosy, leishmaniasis, chiggers, and myiasis. Genital lesions, or any of the protean cutaneous manifestations of AIDS, will require you to take a detailed sexual history.

When assimilating all this information into a single diagnosis always consider the age, sex and ethnic origin of the patient. Malignant melanomas are very rare before puberty. Pemphigoid is principally a problem in the over sixties. Tinea cruris is much commoner in men; nickel dermatitis in women. Keloids are more common in Asian and Afro-Caribbean patients but photosensitivity is less likely in these groups. If your initial diagnosis is quite uncharacteristic of the patient, think again.

Terminology

There is a special terminology used to describe the appearance of skin lesions. It is not essential but it does make descriptions more intelligible:

MACULE

A flat lesion of a different colour from the surrounding skin. There are depigmented macules, erythematous macules, brown macules and so on. Large macules are called 'patches'. The café au lait spot is an example of a pigmented macule or patch.

PAPULE

A small solid skin elevation less than 0.5 cm in diameter. An example would be a lesion of molluscum contagiosum. Elevations larger than this are termed nodules if they are roughly spherical, and plaques if they are flat. Chronic psoriasis typically occurs as large plaques.

VESICLE

A fluid filled papule less than 0.5 cm in diameter. Vesicles commonly occur in contact dermatitis, and pompholyx of the palms where they appear like sago grains. Larger lesions of this type are called bullae. Pemphigoid is a fairly common condition in which large bullae develop. Vesicles and bullae readily rupture and the serum released dries to form a crust.

PUSTULE

A vesicle filled with turbid fluid consisting of leukocytes. Impetigo and varicella are good examples of pustular disorders.

WHEAL

Wheals are areas of transient dermal oedema. Swelling and erythema are seen on the skin surface. Wheals are the classical lesions of urticaria and also follow insect bites.

Descriptive terms like these can be concatenated, for example: 'the rash was maculo-papular' or 'a vesiculo-bullous eruption with secondary crusting'.

Investigations

Never be satisfied with a purely clinical diagnosis if a confirmatory test exists. An account of skin biopsy techniques, histopathology or complex immunological investigations would not be appropriate here. I would however strongly recommend the following procedures.

Fungal identification

Examine skin scrapings from any scaly or approximately annular lesion. A blunt scalpel is suitable for taking the specimen. Material from the active edge of a lesion is placed on a microscope slide and mounted in 10% potassium hydroxide solution. Within 15 minutes or so the skin fragments should have 'cleared' sufficiently for any fungal hyphae present to be clearly visible under the microscope. The presence of candida and the yeast responsible for pityriasis versicolor can also be confirmed in this way. Many hospital microbiology departments will be able to culture fungi from skin, nail or hair samples.

Scabies mites and egg identification

A scabies burrow should be opened up and gently scraped with a needle. The scrapings should be examined under the microscope for mites or eggs. The starting point for this test is the location of an intact burrow. Scratching around at random on an area of excoriated skin will lead to ignominious failure. When instructing an apprehensive, and perhaps slightly hostile, family on de-infestation techniques you can be much more authoritative if irrefutable evidence of the diagnosis is crawling around on a microscope slide!

Wood's light

This is a long-wave ultraviolet lamp which can be most helpful if employed in a darkened room. Wood's light will accentuate pigmentary differences in the epidermis; this property being useful when identifying vitiliginous areas in white skinned individuals in winter. The coral-red fluorescence of erythrasma, or the turquoise-blue of *Microsporum canis* scalp ringworm are both beautiful and diagnostic. Dermatophyte infection of the skin itself does not generate fluorescence but pityriasis versicolor produces a faint yellow coloration. A suitable Wood's light is the UVL 56 Black-ray lamp (UV Products Ltd, Science Park, Milton Road, Cambridge).

Practice points

1 *Extract the maximum information during history taking and use this to reduce the number of possible diagnoses.*
2 *When examining patients: look at individual lesions, the distribution of the rash, and search for additional features of the diagnosis reached.*
3 *Perform a confirmatory test whenever possible. Skin biopsy is often valuable in making a diagnosis but is a specialist procedure.*

2: Topical treatment

Topical preparations normally contain two parts:
1 A vehicle or base, e.g. a cream, paste or gel.
2 An active ingredient, e.g. a corticosteroid or antifungal.
The most suitable combination of vehicle and active ingredients depends on the disease to be treated, and the sites affected.

Vehicles

Vehicles serve to transport an active compound to the required site so that it is released, unaltered, in full potency. Research on the part of the pharmaceutical industry has resulted in the development of many highly efficient and stable vehicles which enable the useful properties of the active ingredients to be fully exploited. My feeling is that 'product liability' considerations now makes the use of personal or extemporaneous mixtures undesirable.

Vehicles can be conveniently classified into lotions, gels, creams, ointments and pastes. There are three classes of materials which such vehicles may contain:
1 *Liquids*: e.g. water, alcohol.
2 *Oils and greases*: mineral, e.g. soft paraffin; animal, e.g. wool fat (lanolin); synthetic, e.g. propylene glycol.
3 *Powders*: e.g. zinc oxide, starch.

Lotions

In their simplest form lotions may be simple chemical solutions, e.g. potassium permanganate solution 0.1%. This is an astringent which seals oozing surfaces. Calamine lotion is a suspension of several insoluble powders, such as zinc carbonate, zinc oxide, ferric oxide and bentonite in a mixture of arachis oil and water. A cooling effect is noted as the aqueous component evaporates and an inert powder is left on the skin. Steroids can be dissolved in mixtures of propylene glycol and ethanol. Such steroid lotions are valuable for treating eczema or psoriasis affecting the scalp.

Gels

These bases are designed to provide the convenience of evaporating bases without the lack of control inherent in 'runny' liquids. Gelling agents convert water or alcohol into a miscible jelly. The gelatinous consistency is lost on contact with the skin and the active ingredient is delivered. Gels are transiently sticky but much less so than creams; they are most valuable when hairy areas are being treated. Benzoyl peroxide containing gels are popular for the treatment of facial acne.

Creams

Creams are emulsions consisting of two immiscible liquids (oil and water) one suspended in the other. Oil-in-water preparations, popularly known as vanishing creams, are the most favoured because they lubricate but do not leave a greasy residue. They are cosmetically acceptable on the face and hands. Examples are aqueous cream and E45 cream (Crookes).

Water-in-oil emulsions, often called moisturizing creams, provide a much more emollient effect leaving a greasier residue but helping to promote skin suppleness. They are popular bases for preparations designed to treat dry eczemas or ichthyosis; an example is oily cream.

Creams are often quite complicated mixtures. Stabilizers may be necessary to prevent the emulsion separating into its two component parts. Because creams have an aqueous phase preservatives, like parabens, chlorocresol or sorbic acid, must be incorporated to prevent the growth of moulds and bacteria. Lanolin is a liquid obtained by the fractionation of sheep's wool fat. This substance and its derivatives blend well with mineral and vegetable oils and are popular emulsifiers in topical formulations. Both lanolin and the preservatives may produce allergic reactions.

Ointments

Ointments are thicker than creams and contain no water; such bases are not used sufficiently. They are the most effective means of promoting water retention within the epidermis and thus increasing the penetration of active ingredients. Ointments leave the skin feeling greasy but this is acceptable for the initial treatment of chronically dry and inflexible skin. White soft paraffin is a mixture of semisolid hydrocarbons and is a decolorized petroleum distillate. It is a common constituent of ointments and is a useful vehicle for medicaments which are insoluble in water, for example coal tar.

Mixtures of lanolin, hard, soft and liquid paraffins produce the various types of hydrophobic or non-emulsifying ointments. One example of a non-emulsifying preparation is 'simple ointment'. The water soluble or hydrophilic ointments have the useful additional property of being washable in warm water. A widely used example is emulsifying ointment which contains emulsifying wax in addition to soft and liquid paraffin.

Pastes

Pastes result from the addition of powders to an ointment. One example, Lassar's paste, contains starch, zinc oxide and salicyclic acid in soft paraffin. Pastes are valuable as protective preparations on or around damaged skin, like the napkin area in babies. They can also be formulated to remain solid at body temperature. This is useful if a drug, like dithranol, is to be applied to a well-demarcated lesion without spreading to surrounding skin. Pastes cannot be removed easily by washing but should be gently rubbed off with oil on cotton wool.

Newer ingredients

Manufacturers are constantly devising new bases and ingredients in an attempt to obtain useful combinations of properties. Steroids are soluble in propylene glycol. Water and gelling agents can convert this solution into a miscible gel. Addition of stearic acid and cetostearyl alcohol can convert the solution into a semisolid cream. This FAPG (fatty alcohols propylene glycol) cream is a useful vehicle with some intrinsic antiseptic properties but it may cause stinging and burning. Macrogol esters are condensation products prepared from fatty alcohols and ethylene oxide. Cetomacrogol 1000 is an example of this group. Macrogols are used as solvents for drugs which are relatively insoluble in water. They are useful stabilizers in emulsions.

Quantities of topical preparations to be prescribed

It takes approximately 25 g of a cream to cover the skin surface of an adult. It follows that 250 g of a cream is a reasonable amount for a 2 week supply, although clearly some preparations, like very potent topical steroids, are never prescribed on this scale. For the same period 25–50 g would be sufficient to treat both hands or the groin and 200 ml would be a suitable supply of scalp lotion. Patients are apt to lose confidence in their doctor if the quantity of medication prescribed is totally at variance with the instructions they have been given.

Practice points

1 *Creams and gels are popular vehicles but occasional patients will become allergic to the preservatives they contain.*
2 *Ointments and pastes are less cosmetically acceptable but have valuable properties.*
3 *Prescribe quantities of medication appropriate for the course of treatment you intend.*

Topical steroids

Hydrocortisone, the first topically effective corticosteroid, was introduced in the late 1950s. The subsequent explosive development of this class of drugs has tended to obscure the usefulness of the parent compound. More recent topical steroids show increased efficacy and potency but are associated with far more unwanted actions.

Because of their powerful anti-inflammatory effect topical

steroids are an essential part of the management of many skin disorders. Used indiscriminately they can do great harm. Table 2.1 gives some guidance on their use.

Table 2.1   The response of dermatoses to topical steroids

Usually respond	May respond	Never respond	Contraindicated
Eczema	Alopecia areata	Ichthyosis	Acne
Contact	Vitiligo	Urticaria	Rosacea
dermatitis		Neoplasms	Infections
Flexural psoriasis			Leg ulcers
Lichen planus			
Discoid lupus			
erythematosus			

Modifications to the structure of hydrocortisone by halogenation has increased the anti-inflammatory activity. Many of the more powerful topical steroids are 'fluorinated'. There are however potent topical steroids which are not fluorinated, e.g. budesonide (Preferid: Gist-Brocades).

After application the rate of penetration of a steroid into the stratum corneum is greater the more hydrated the keratin. Thus the regular use of emollients, such as emulsifying ointment, increases the absorption of a topical steroid considerably. Penetration into the living cell is conversely enhanced by increased lipid solubility, a quality conferred by esterification.

The vehicles for the many topical steroid preparations have been developed bearing in mind the physical chemistry of the materials used. Any subsequent alteration of the solubilities and partition coefficients may profoundly effect the clinical effectiveness of the steroid. The practice of users adding diluents or additives is unsound. The manufacturer's base is best and if diluted preparations are required it is advisable to use those available off the shelf (e.g. Betnovate RD: Glaxo; Synalar 1 in 4: ICI). The adddition of tar or salicylic acid to a steroid hastens isomerization to a less active form. The only exceptions to this principle are where a manufacturer has taken great care to stabilize the compound, for example, betamethasone diproprionate and 3% salicylic acid ointment (Diprosalic: Kirby-Warrick).

Clinical uses

Topical steroids are classified according to their potency (Table 2.2). Become familiar with a small number of products from each group. Select the preparation most appropriate for the clinical situation and never use a more potent steroid than is necessary.

Table 2.2 The classification of a selection of topical steroids by potency

Group	Type	Approved name	Manufacturer's name
4	Weak	Hydrocortisone	Efcortelan
3	Moderate	Clobetasone butyrate	Eumovate
		Flurandrenolone	Haelan
2	Potent	Betamethasone valerate	Betnovate
		Hydrocortisone butyrate	Locoid
		Betamethasone proprionate	Diprosone
		Fluocinolone acetonide	Synalar
1	Very potent	Clobetasol propionate	Dermovate
		Diflucortolone valerate	Nerisone Forte

Hydrocortisone preparations are the oldest, weakest and safest of the topical steroids. The delivery of hydrocortisone can be made more efficient by increasing skin hydration. The addition of 10% urea to the vehicle will achieve this. Examples are Alphaderm (Norwich Eaton) and Calmurid HC (Pharmacia). These preparations are suitable for all sites and there is nothing to be gained by further dilution.

Several years ago in the UK hydrocortisone 1% became available as an over-the-counter preparation for a restricted group of indications (Table 2.3).

The more potent topical steroids are valuable in the treatment of active and inflammatory dermatoses particularly eczema, contact dermatitis and lichen planus. There is rarely any need to use topical steroids more than twice daily. Exudative or

Table 2.3   Use of over-the-counter hydrocortisone

Indications	Irritant dermatitis
	Contact allergic dermatitis
	Insect bite reactions
Contraindications	Children under 10 years
	Use on face, eye or anogenital region
	Use on broken or infected skin
Precautions	1 week maximum period of use

weeping lesions should be treated with a cream. Dry or lichenified areas require a greasy ointment base.

Initially it may be necessary to control a disease with a potent steroid, for example Betnovate ointment, but subsequently a diluted preparation (Betnovate RD ointment) may be sufficient. The face and flexures are very susceptible to steroid damage, whereas the scalp and palms are relatively resistant. The skin of children is more prone to damage than that of adults.

Side-effects of topical steroids

Although systemic absorption of steroids occurs after application no clinically significant hypothalamic−pituitary−adrenal suppression develops in the vast majority of patients. The notable exception to this principle are babies who have a large surface area relative to their weight. Iatrogenic Cushing's syndrome can follow potent topical steroid application at this age and only group 3 and 4 steroids should be prescribed.

In practice the adverse actions of topical steroids are dominated by local side-effects; the stronger the steroid the more likely are these unwanted effects to develop (Table 2.4).

Additives

Topical steroids are commonly combined with anti-microbial agents for the management of infected dermatoses such as flexural eczema and psoriasis. They are certainly not indicated in primary bacterial or fungal infections of the skin. Examples

Table 2.4 Local side-effects of topical steroid therapy

Adverse effect	Comments
Local infection	Commonly bacterial folliculitis
Exacerbation of infection	e.g. worsening of tinea cruris
Atrophic changes	Striae or bruising
Perioral dermatitis	Facial erythema, pustules and papules
Acneiform eruption	Comedones and papules
Leucoderma	After occlusion

of such preparations are Haelan-C, Propaderm, and Betnovate-N. The additives employed include:
- 3% clioquinol (-C): a yellow broad-spectrum antiseptic
- 3% chlortetracycline (-A): a broad-spectrum antibiotic
- 0.5% neomycin (-N): an anti-staphylococcal antibiotic

Dermovate-NN contains neomycin and nystatin. These agents combined with a topical steroid are also found in Tri-Adcortyl cream (Squibb). Hydrocortisone has recently become a popular additive to antifungal and antibiotic preparations. Its presence may be indicated by the suffix -HC or -H, e.g. Nystaform HC, Canestan HC or Fucidin H.

Practice points

1 *Before prescribing ensure that the disease is steroid responsive.*
2 *Use the weakest possible steroid in the most appropriate base.*
3 *Never used a combined preparation if any constituent used alone would be equally effective.*

Antimicrobial agents

NEOMYCIN

This antibiotic is effective against the staphylococci and Gram-negative organism. It is used alone (neomycin cream) but a lack of effect against the haemolytic streptococcus has resulted in the popularity of combinations of neomycin with bacitracin, e.g. Cicatrin cream (Calmic). Neomycin is widely recognized as a cause of contact sensitivity. Framycetin and gentamicin have similar spectra and side-effects.

FUSIDIC ACID AND SODIUM FUSIDATE

This valuable systemic antibiotic has a limited spectrum but is highly effective against the staphylococci, including many penicillin resistant strains. Fusidic acid penetrates the skin well. It is available as a gel or cream (Fucidin: Leo) and might have a place in the treatment of impetigo.

TETRACYCLINE, CLINDAMYCIN AND ERYTHROMYCIN

Several preparations are available for the treatment of acne; they are applied twice daily for 3 months.
- tetracycline 0.22% (Topicycline: Norwich Eaton)
- clindamycin 10 mg/ml (Dalacin T: Upjohn)
- erythromycin 2% (Stiemycin: Stiefel)

MUPIROCIN

This novel broad-spectrum antibacterial agent was previously known as pseudomonic acid. It is supplied as 2% mupirocin in a water soluble base (Bactroban ointment: Beecham). Mupirocin has a broad-spectrum of activity; bacterial resistance and allergic reactions are rare. In every respect, except possibly that of price, it is an ideal topical antibacterial agent.

POLYMYXIN AND BACITRACIN

Polyfax ointment (Calmic) is a combination of these antibiotics. It is clean, rarely sensitizes, and is effective against Gram-negative and positive organisms.

CHLORHEXIDINE GLUCONATE

This is particularly active against Gram-positive bacteria and is available in many forms. A 1% cream (Hibitane: ICI) is useful for the treatment of impetigo. A 0.5% solution in 70%

alcohol is used for skin cleansing prior to minor surgery. Hibiscrub (ICI) is a detergent solution containing 4% chlorhexidine used in the treatment of acne. Chlorhexidine is inactivated by alkaline soaps.

IODINE

Iodine has always been an effective if messy antiseptic. In its elemental form it stained and caused allergic reactions. The complex of iodine and povidone retains the antiseptic qualities but unwanted features are much reduced. This tincture is also washable. Betadine 10% ointment (Napp) is suitable for impetigo and leg ulcers. A paint, and a 7.5% scalp and skin cleanser are also available.

HYDROXYQUINOLONES

These are widely used as topical antiseptics and are frequently combined with steroid preparations (e.g. Haelan-C). They have an antibacterial and some antifungal activity. A clioquinol cream (Vioform: Ciba) is available. Hydroxyquinolone impregnated paste bandages (e.g. Quinaband: Seton) are used in the management of leg ulcers and infected eczema of the limbs. The disadvantages of all hydroxyquinolones is the yellowish staining they produce.

ROSANILINE DYES

Rosaniline dyes are active against *Candida albicans* and Grampositive organisms but have always been unpopular because of the staining they produce. They may be toxic to regenerating epithelium. Gentian (Crystal) Violet 0.5% and Brilliant Green are still occasionally used for the treatment of leg ulcers but I believe that these traditional dyes are now decidedly obsolescent.

POTASSIUM PERMANGANATE

This is an astringent and antiseptic. It is valuable in the treatment of weeping and infected eczemas particularly of the

hands and feet. It is best used in 1 : 8000 to 1 : 10 000 dilution.
It is usually supplied as 500 ml of 0.1% potassium permanganate solution which should be diluted approximately 8–10
times before use. Permitabs (Bioglan) 400 mg, one per 4 litres
of water are a convenient alternative.

HYPOCHLORITES

Chlorinated solutions have long been popular in the cleansing
of ulcers and wounds. An example is Eusol solution (chlorinated
lime and boric acid) which has 0.25% available chlorine. Eusol
is often employed in a 50% mix with liquid paraffin to prevent
dressing adherence. There is experimental evidence that hypo-
chlorites are toxic to granulation tissue and their use in the
management of leg ulcers should be abandoned.

ANTIVIRAL AGENTS

Herpes virus infections can be treated with two specific agents,
idoxuridine (IDU) and acyclovir. IDU is incorporated into viral
DNA; this apparently makes the viral DNA chain more likely
to break thus inhibiting replication. For dermatological use it
is supplied as a 5% solution in dimethylsulphoxide (DMSO).
(Iduridin: Nordic; Herpid: Boehringer; Virudox; Bioglan). The
vehicle accelerates absorption through the skin but is irritant
and may cause transient stinging. DMSO excreted in the
breath has a garlic-like smell. The lotion should be applied
4–6 times daily for the first 4 days of the attack. Acyclovir 5%
cream (Zovirax: Wellcome) is available in 2 and 10 g tubes.
The preparation should be applied five times daily for 5 days.

ANTIFUNGAL AGENTS

The treatment of fungal and yeast infections has been simplified
by the introduction of the imidazoles. Imidazoles have a broad-
spectrum and are effective against the dermatophytes (ringworm producing fungi), yeasts and even some bacteria. Since
the development of the first, clotrimazole, there have been a
number of these broad-spectrum agents synthesized. All are
available in cream form:

- clotrimazole 1% (Canesten: Bayer) 20, 50 g
- sulconazole 1% (Exelderm: ICI) 30 g
- miconazole 2% (Daktarin: Janssen) 15, 30 g
- ketoconazole 2% (Nizoral: Janssen) 30 g
- econazole 1% (Ecostatin: Squibb) 15, 30 g (or Pevaryl: Cilag 30 g)

One of the few weaknesses of the imidazoles is their inability to penetrate nail plates. A new imidazole, tioconazole (Trosyl nail solution: Pfizer), has been formulated in an undecylenic acid vehicle. This preparation gives high concentrations in nail plates and may permit the cure of tinea unguium without the need for systemic agents. Toe-web fungus infection may be surprisingly resistant to any treatment.

The imidazoles' spectrum of activity includes the yeasts *Pityrosporum orbiculare* (the cause of pityriasis versicolor) and *Candida albicans*. Econazole lotion (Pevaryl: Cilag) is particularly useful for nail bed infections. Miconazole oral gel 5–10 ml four times daily is a pleasant orange-flavoured preparation for treating oral candidiasis. Nystatin is still highly effective against this yeast. Preparations available include:

- nystatin 10 000 U/g cream or gel (Nystan: Princeton)
- nystan pastilles (Princeton), suck one four times daily

Insecticides

Substances that are widely used for the treatment of scabies include:

- benzyl benzoate
- monosulfiram
- lindane (gammabenzene hexachloride)
- malathion

Benzyl benzoate 25% solution is now obselescent. Its disadvantages are the stinging it produces and the fact that three applications are required. In contrast only a single application of 1% Lindane cream or lotion (Lorexane: ICI: Quellada: Stafford Miller) is required although a second treatment, one week after the first, is often advised.

In many respects Lindane is an ideal treatment being effective, non-stinging and easy to apply. It is, however, a highly lipid soluble organochlorine insecticide and some doubts have been expressed over its safety during pregnancy and in infants. Certainly transcutaneous absorption does take place after application and the drug is potentially neurotoxic. I am not convinced that actual damage has ensued following *the correct use* of the product. It seems sensible to minimize absorption in susceptible groups; this involves dispensing with any pretreatment bath, washing the material off after 6 hours and not proceeding with further applications without specific medical advice.

Monosulfiram (Tetmosol: ICI) is effective and is often stated to be the preferred preparation in children. It is presented as an alcoholic solution that requires dilution with two or three parts of water before use. Unfortunately the solution is inflammable and two or three applications may be necessary. In adults the possibility of an alcohol initiated disulfiram-reaction may be a problem. Crotamiton cream 10% (Eurax: Geigy) is useful for treating the persistent scabies nodules that develop on the penis and scrotum of adult males, and the axillae of children.

Malathion preparations are effective against the scabies mite but in the UK are mainly reserved for treating lice. Both malathion and carbaryl are anti-cholinesterases. They lead to a build up of acetylcholine in the louse. Abnormal discharge of nerve impulses leads to fatal discoordinated movements. A number of preparations are available. Lotions should be applied to the scalp and allowed to dry naturally. Naked lights and hot hair dryers should be avoided because alcohol containing bases are inflammable and the active compounds thermolabile. The preparations are very irritating to the eyes and should not be used carelessly. After 12 hours the hair should be thoroughly washed and fine-tooth combed.

- malathion 0.5%

Suleo-M	(International)	alcoholic
Prioderm	(Napp)	alcoholic
Derbac-M	(International)	aqueous

- carbaryl 0.5%

Suleo-C	(International)	alcoholic
Carylderm	(Napp)	alcoholic

Practice points

1 *Avoid topical antibiotics with a valuable systemic role.*
2 *Nystatin is effective against* Candida albicans *but it lacks the broad spectrum of the imidazoles.*
3 *Scabies and head-lice are usually diagnostic not therapeutic problems.*

Tar and dithranol

Tar preparations

Tars are the products of the destructive distillation of wood or coal. Crude coal tar is produced by distilling bituminous coal in the absence of oxygen. It consists of thousands of hydrocarbons including phenols, cresols and naphthalenes. Strong coal tar solution is a filtered alcoholic extract which is incorporated into many tar pastes and ointments. Tar has antiproliferative, antipruritic and antiseptic actions. A wood tar, cade oil, is still occasionally employed, particularly in medicated shampoos. Topical steroids have not superseded all the functions of tar. The main indication is the treatment of psoriasis and eczema. The 'cruder' the tar preparation, the more effective it is. Examples of widely used tar preparations are:
1 Coal tar paste. Strong coal tar solution 7.5%.
2 Coal tar and salicylic acid ointment.
3 Gelcotar (Quinoderm) 50 g. Strong coal tar solution 5%, pine tar 5%.
4 Alphosyl cream (Stafford-Miller) 75 g. 5% coal tar extract.
  Tar creams and lotions can be applied to the scalp and washed out with a tar based shampoo. Widely used products are Alphosyl lotion and Polytar liquid (Stiefel).

DITHRANOL (*USA Anthralin*)

Dithranol is a synthetic tricyclic quinone. Hydroxyanthracene derivatives like dithranol have been used for the treatment of psoriasis for over 100 years although the therapeutic action is still uncertain. It is possible that dithranol has a cytotoxic action resulting from the inhibition of DNA replication. Alternatively highly reactive peroxide and free hydroxyl radicals, generated after application, may inhibit phagocyte chemotaxis and lymphocyte function. Whatever the mechanism the excessive epidermal proliferation in psoriasis is slowed and consequently the clinical condition improves.

A dithranol containing cream or paste is applied accurately to the plaques of psoriasis. The concentration of dithranol is gradually increased until the desired effect is obtained. All dithranol preparations cause some staining of the skin and clothes. An irritant dermatitis can result from treatment with high concentrations and the material must be kept out of the eyes. Examples of preparations available are:

1 Dithranol 0.1–2.0% in Lassar's paste. A traditional paste which needs oil for removal.

2 Dithrocream 0.1, 0.25, 0.5, 1.0, 2.0% (Dermal) 90 g. Washable cream. Care must be taken to prevent spread to uninvolved skin.

3 Psoradrate cream 0.1, 0.2, 0.4% (Norwich Eaton) 30 g : 100 g. Contains urea which may help to remove resistent scale.

Practice points

1 *Topical steroids have not superseded all the functions of tars and dithranol.*

2 *Dithranol and tar preparations are too irritating for flexural use and should be kept out of the eyes.*

Other topical agents

SALICYLIC ACID

The main action of salicylic acid is to soften scale. In high concentration it will macerate callosities; for example:

1 Salicylic acid oint 2% BNF 50 g.

2 Keralyt gel 6% (Bristol-Myers) 55 g, for use in ichthyosis and localized hyperkeratoses.

Salicylic acid is also a component of various wart paints; for example:

1 Salactol (Dermal) 10 ml; salicylic and lactic acid in collodion.
2 Salactac (Dermal) 8 ml; a viscous gel containing salicylic acid 12% and lactic acid 4%.
3 Cuplex (S&N) 5 g. Gel containing copper acetate and lactic acid.

UREA

A hydrating and keratolytic agent. In high concentrations (40%) it is used by dermatologists and chiropodists to soften nails made dystrophic by fungal invasion. The damaged nail plates are then easy to remove. Unfortunately at the time of writing no commercial preparation of this type is available. In lower concentration (10%) it is used in a cream base to treat ichthyosis (e.g. Calmurid: Pharmacia; Aquadrate: Norwich Eaton) and to enhance the penetration of hydrocortisone (Alphaderm: Norwich Eaton; Calmurid HC: Pharmacia).

BENZOYL PEROXIDE

Benzoyl peroxide is extensively used in prescribable and over-the-counter acne preparations. It has peeling and antiseptic properties. Care has be taken to avoid an irritant reaction. When first applied patients should be recommended to use benzoyl peroxide at a low concentration for 4 hours only, after which time it should be washed off. Within 7–10 days it should be possible to leave the preparation on all day. The concentration of benzoyl peroxide should then be increased until the maximum benefit is obtained. Washes, lotions, gels and creams are all available and should be used according to patient preference, for example:

1 Acetoxyl 2.5, 5% (Stiefel) 40 g; Aqueous acetone gel base.
2 Acnidazil (Janssen) 20 g; benzoyl peroxide 5% and miconazole 2%.
3 Panoxyl 2.5, 5, 10% (Stiefel) 40 g; aqueous alcohol base.
4 Quinoderm 5, 10% (Quinoderm Ltd) 50 g cream and lotion, also contains hydroxyquinoline.

Sunscreens

A sunscreen is a substance which when applied to the skin will either absorb or reflect the sun's harmful rays which are mainly those of wavelength 290−320 nm (ultraviolet B). The absorbers are chemical agents like PABA (*para*-amino benzoic acid) PABA esters, benzophenones, cinnamates, salicylates and anthranilates. The physical reflectors are used particularly for those patients reactive to long-wave ultraviolet and visible light (Table 2.5). They contain titanium dioxide and/or zinc oxide but because these materials are opaque they are less cosmetically acceptable.

Table 2.5 Indications for regular sunscreen use

Photosensitivity
Facial vitiligo
Albinism
Red hair or a very fair complexion

The degree of protection afforded by a particular preparation is designated by its sun protection factor (SPF) (Table 2.6). This is the ratio of the least amount of sunlight (or more correctly UVB) required to cause minimal skin redness with the sunscreen to that required when no screen is present. The higher the factor the better the protection.

Patients should be given clear instructions on the use of the sunscreen (see Table 2.7 for sunscreens that are available). In general they should be applied evenly and generously to exposed

Table 2.6 Effectiveness of sunscreens

Degree of protection	SPF	Clinical use
Minimal	2−4	Those who tan readily
Moderate	4−6	Those who tan gradually
Extra sun protection	6−8	Fair or actinic damaged skin
Maximal protection	15−23	Vitiligo, photodermatoses or previous skin cancer

Table 2.7   Sunscreens currently available

Manufacturer's name	Approved name	SPF
Uvistat	4% Mexenone cream (60 g)	4
Spectraban 4	Padimate 3.2% lotion (150 ml)	4
Spectraban 15	Padimate 3.2%, aminobenzoic acid 5% lotion (50 ml)	15
Roc 15 A & B	Methoxycinnamate and zinc oxide cream	15
Coppertone 15	Padimate 7%, oxybenzone 3% lotion	15
Coppertone 23	Padimate 2.5%, oxybenzone 3%, parsol MCX 7.5% lotion	23

areas of skin. Two or three applications each day are normally sufficient; reapplication after swimming is sensible.

Topical chemotherapy

5-Fluorouracil is a 'fraudulent' nucleotide which is available as a 5% cream (Efudix: Roche). It is used to treat skin malignancies and pre-malignancies like Bowen's disease, actinic keratoses and superficial basal cell carcinomas. The lesion to be treated is cleaned of debris and the cream applied daily. Usually this will produce a marked inflammatory reaction of the lesion but not in the surrounding normal skin. A month's treatment will normally complete destruction and a topical antiseptic can then be applied until healing takes place. The course can be repeated if required. In the UK Efudix is at present not available outside hospitals.

Podophyllin is an intensely irritant compound extracted from the rhizomes of the Indian herbs *Podophyllum peltatum* and *P. emodi*. The intermittent application of a 25% solution in alcohol or benzoin tincture is employed for the treatment of genital warts where it apparently acts as a cytotoxic. It is contra-indicated in pregnant women because of possible teratogenicity and neurotoxicity. Podophyllin should be applied accurately to each lesion under direct vision, preferably by a doctor or nurse.

Recently two preparations of 0.5% podophyllotoxin, the pharmacologically active constituent of podophyllum resin, have been introduced. These are Condyline (Gist-Brocades) and Warticon (Kabi). The preparations should be applied twice daily for 3 days. The treatment can be repeated after 1 week if required. Podophyllotoxin is less irritating than the parent extract and self-treatment is reasonable for sensible male patients with penile warts.

Posalfilin (Norgine) is a mixture of salicylic acid 25% and podophyllum resin 20% in an ointment base. It can be applied to plantar warts two to three times weekly under plaster. Unfortunately it may produce a profound irritant dermatitis and I cannot recommend it.

Contact dermatitis to skin preparations

Topical preparations consist of an active ingredient suspended in a base which may be a complicated mixture of water, oils, preservatives and emulsifiers. Cosmetic creams are very similar. They contain no active ingredient but include perfumes, dyes, and ultraviolet light absorbers. Any part of this formulation may produce a contact dermatitis. Those most commonly encountered are given in Table 2.8, but the list is by no means exhaustive.

Table 2.8 Sensitizers in topical preparations

Active agents	Neomycin
	Bacitracin
	Framycetin
	Gentamicin
	Quinolines, e.g. vioform, chinoform, clioquinol
Base ingredients	Lanolin
	Propylene glycol
	Cetostearyl alcohol
	Fragrances
	Butylated hydroxyanisole
Preservatives	Chlorocresol
	Hydroxybenzoates (parabens)
	Formaldehyde releasers (Dowicil 200, bronopol)
	Ethylenediamine
	Sorbic acid

The current *British National Formulary* (BNF) lists the ingredients of many topical preparations. The labelling of such products with all their ingredients is usual in many parts of the world but is not yet obligatory in the UK.

Practice points

If you suspect the development of a medicament dermatitis because a treated skin rash is deteriorating:

1 *Change to an ointment rather than a cream.*

2 *Change the active ingredient and use the simplest possible vehicle, e.g. soft paraffin.*

3: Systemic treatment

Antimicrobial agents

Penicillin, flucloxacillin and erythromycin

These antibiotics are indicated for the treatment of skin infecions such as erysipelas and impetigo. Benzyl penicillin is still the drug of choice in erysipelas; broader spectrum agents are nothing like so effective. Erythromycin is cheap and safe; most staphylococcal infections contracted in the community are sensitive.

Tetracyclines

The tetracyclines are the first-line agents for treating moderately severe acne, rosacea, and peri-oral dermatitis. Their mechanism of action is not fully understood. Because of the dental damage produced tetracyclines should not be prescribed in pregnancy nor to children under twelve. Like all broad spectrum antibiotics the use of tetracycline may encourage candida super-infection of the bowel or vagina. Minocycline (Minocin: Lederle) is now very widely used to treat acne. It is perhaps more active than oxytetracycline and the absorption of the drug is less influenced by dietary factors. These advantages do not in my view compensate for its much greater cost; minocycline may produce reversible bluish-grey pigmentation of skin and acne scars.

Metronidazole

This agent has high activity against anaerobic bacteria (especially *Bacteroides fragilis*) and trichomonas but is mainly used by dermatologists as an alternative to tetracycline in rosacea. If highly offensive leg ulcers are infected with bacteroides species then metronidazole may reduce the odour. Metronidazole may cause an 'antabuse-like' interaction with alcohol.

Antifungal drugs

Griseofulvin

Griseofulvin (Fulcin: ICI; Grisovin: Glaxo) has been used to treat dermatophyte infections for many years. After absorption the drug is incorporated into developing keratin where it prevents further invasion of keratin by damaging actively growing hyphae. Eventually all the infected keratin is shed resulting in clinical cure. This process may not progress to completion in toe-nails. Griseofulvin is contra-indicated in pregnancy and can cause gastro-intestinal upsets or leucopenia. It is not indicated in trivial infections which respond to topical therapy alone. The spectrum of activity of griseofulvin does not include the yeasts; it is therefore of no value in the treatment of candidiasis or pityriasis versicolor.

Ketoconazole and itraconazole

The spectrum of the orally effective imidazole ketoconazole (Nizoral: Janssen) includes ringworm producing fungi, and yeasts. It is usually given in a dose of 200 mg daily. It has one rare, but serious, side-effect that of drug induced hepatitis. This problem is dose independent and can be irreversible if undiagnosed and untreated. The risks are believed to be greater in the elderly and those on prolonged courses of treatment. Short 10–14 day courses of treatment, such as might be given to extensive pityriasis versicolor, are almost certainly safe. Ketoconazole should be avoided for long-term treatment of nail plate infections.

Itraconazole (Sporanox:Janssen) is effective against *Candida albicans* and the organisms responsible for ringworm and pityriasis versicolor. It is best absorbed if taken immediately after food. Itraconazole is not considered safe in pregnancy, or in those with a history of liver disease. It is a member of a new class of imidazole derivatives called triazoles. Like the imidazoles they inhibit the fungal demethylation of lanesterol to form ergosterol, an important constituent of the fungal cell membrane.

Antiviral drugs

Acyclovir (Zovirax: Wellcome) is active against herpes simplex and varicella zoster virus. Phosphorylation of the drug to the active compound acyclovir triphosphate is dependent on a viral coded enzyme, thymidine kinase. The active compound then inhibits viral DNA polymerase. Effectively viral DNA synthesis is prevented but mammalian cellular function continues unhindered. The drug has very low toxicity.

Used systemically acyclovir is indicated in eczema herpeticum and severe herpes simplex in neonates or the immunocompromised. An adult dose would be 200 mg 6-hourly for 5 days initially. As little acyclovir as 200 mg 12-hourly may prevent recurrent attacks of herpes simplex. Continuous treatment of this type would normally be considered only if the patient is suffering frequent relapses of severe genital herpes, or herpes induced erythema multiforme. In herpes zoster the recommended regime is 800 mg five times daily for 7 days beginning as soon as possible after diagnosis. Treatment with acyclovir reduces acute pain and produces a modest reduction in healing time. It is expensive and has not yet been proven to reduce the incidence of post-herpetic neuralgia.

Zidovudine (Retrovir: Wellcome) inhibits the viral enzyme reverse transcriptase. It prevents the retrovirus responsible for AIDS from replicating but does not actually remove the infection.

Antihistamines

These drugs act as competitive antagonists to histamine at its receptor sites (H_1 − bronchial mucosa: H_2 − gastric mucosa). The skin contains both H_1 and H_2 receptors. The significance of this pharmacological fact is uncertain although it has led to the use of combinations of H_1 blockers (like chlorpheniramine) and H_2 blockers (like cimetidine or ranitidine) in urticaria. Some anti-histamines have additional anti-serotonin or anticholinergic effects.

Patients receiving conventional antihistamines should be warned not to mix them with alcohol and to exercise caution in driving or operating machinery. In general the doses of antihistamines are slowly increased until either therapeutic or unwanted effects occur. If one drug fails another, of a different chemical class, should be tried.

Over the last 10 years new antihistamines have been developed which have a purely peripheral action and do not cross the blood−brain barrier. Non-sedating antihistamines are valuable in urticaria where sedative side-effects are a major nuisance. They are less helpful if a central effect is needed, for example an anti-pruritic effect in atopic eczema. It is doubtful if any antihistamine has overall superiority to any other but they differ in their duration of action, cost, and the incidence of anti-cholinergic and sedative side-effects.

Trimeprazine and hydroxyzine

Trimeprazine (Vallergan: May & Baker) and hydroxyzine (Atarax: Pfizer) have sedative and anxiolytic properties. They are popular and safe for treating pruritus in childhood.

Cyproheptadine

This antihistamine (Periactin: MSD) has the reputation of being more effective in the 'physical' urticarias.

Terfenadine and astemizole

Terfenadine (Triludan: Merrell Dow) is used in doses of 60−120 mg twice daily. It is probably the most widely prescribed of the non-sedating antihistamines. Astemizole (Hismanal: Janssen) is also non-sedating. It is given in a convenient 10 mg nightly dose. Astemizole is also a weak serotonin antagonist but has a relatively slow onset of action. Like cyproheptadine it has the interesting side-effect of increasing appetite and promoting weight gain.

New agents

Other non-sedating antihistamines recently introduced in the UK are acrivastine (Semprex: Calmic), loratadine (Clarityn:

Kirby Warrick) and cetirizine (Zirtek: Allen and Hansburys), which is a metabolite of hydroxyzine.

Retinoids

Vitamin A was originally used in the 1920s to treat scaly skin disorders but the benefits were inconstant and the drug was found to be hepatotoxic and neurotoxic. Many retinoid derivatives have subsequently been synthesized and two are widely used in the UK.

Etretinate (Tigason: Roche; *USA Tegison*) has been employed in the management of ichthyosis, psoriasis and other disorders of keratinization. The dose for an adult is 25–100 mg daily. The duration of treatment depends on response. Isotretinoin (Roaccutane: Roche; *USA Accutane*) is probably the most effective agent for the treatment of severe acne. It seems to work by causing sebaceous gland atrophy. The most effective schedule is 1 mg/Kg body weight per day and 3–4 months continuous treatment is normally required.

Retinoids are relatively expensive and have a high incidence of side-effects such as cheilitis, blepheritis and mild reversible hair loss. There are some more significant long-term side-effects like hyperlipidaemia and skeletal damage. The major practical difficulty is the teratogenicity of these drugs. It is not safe to conceive whilst taking etretinate because of the very high incidence of associated congenital abnormalities. A reservoir of etretinate forms in body fat stores and therefore the hazard remains for 2 years after the drug has been discontinued. With isotretinoin the interval before safe conception is at least 4 weeks. In the UK the retinoids are available for purely hospital use and would normally be prescribed to fertile women only if they had a negative pregnancy test and were prepared to take an oral contraceptive.

Cytotoxics and related agents

Azathioprine (Imuran: Wellcome) is an immunosuppressant widely used to treat autoimmune diseases. It is used as a steroid sparing agent in the management of pemphigus, pemphigoid, SLE and dermato-myositis. The drug is metabolized to mercaptopurine. Since this product is further metabolized by the enzyme xanthine oxidase it follows that the dose of azathioprine must be reduced during concurrent treatment with allopurinol. The major side-effect is bone marrow suppression but nausea and hepatic damage may also result from its use.

The folic acid antagonist methotrexate (Lederle) is probably the most effective anti-psoriatic agent. Hepatotoxicity, marrow suppression and peripheral neuropathy have been associated with its use. Methotrexate may produce widespread and painful epidermal necrosis and ulceration; less seriously it may produce lip ulceration, photosensitivity or a folate responsive macrocytic anaemia. Methotrexate is mainly removed from the blood by renal clearance; any impairment of renal function greatly increases the likelihood of adverse reactions. There are also important drug interactions with trimethoprim and non-steroidal anti-inflammatory drugs (NSAID). The major side-effect, liver damage, can develop insidiously despite normal liver function tests. Fortunately a single weekly dose of methotrexate (e.g. 5–20 mg orally or intramuscularly) is much less likely to produce liver toxicity than a smaller daily dose and is equally effective in the treatment of psoriasis.

Despite all these hazards many severely disabled and resistant psoriatic patients have their disease well controlled for years with methotrexate therapy. The only possible drugs to emerge as rivals are hyroxyurea (Hydrea: Squibb) and, more recently cyclosporin (Sandimmun: Sandoz). Cyclosporin is an immunosuppressive fungal metabolite widely used after organ transplantation surgery. It is expensive and has many toxic side-effects including hypertension and nephrotoxicity but it is effective in controlling severe psoriasis. The use of this drug is likely to increase within the next few years.

Hormones

Cyproterone acetate is an anti-androgen which blocks androgen receptors and decreases androgen synthesis. In the contraceptive preparation Dianette (Schering) 2 mg of the drug is combined with 35 mg of ethinyloestradiol. The oestrogen is essential to prevent conception and feminization of the male fetus. Dianette is indicated in the treatment of resistant acne in females and may have a slightly beneficial effect on mild idiopathic hirsutism. In common with other anovulants there may be a slightly increased risk of arterial embolism and venous thrombosis.

Antimalarials

Chloroquine and hydroxychloroquine were originally antimalarial drugs. They were adopted by rheumatologists for the treatment of rheumatoid disease. In high doses and over long periods they can cause retinal damage which may be irreversible. Dermatologists use chloroquine to treat discoid lupus erythematosus, cutaneous sarcoidosis and several rarer disorders. Used in doses of 200 mg (hydroxychloroquine or chloroquine sulphate) twice daily or 250 mg (chloroquine phosphate) twice daily for less than 6 months retinal damage is unlikely. Other side-effects include nausea and the exacerbation of psoriasis.

Lipids

Maxepa capsules (Duncan Flockhart) contain 1 g of a marine fish oil. The active constituents are eicosapentaenoic acid and docosahexaenoic acid. Initially the preparation was introduced for the reduction of plasma triglycerides in patients with hypertriglyceridaemia. The consumption of fish is believed to account for the relatively low incidence of ischaemic heart disease in Greenland Eskimos. Regular consumption of Maxepa produces a modest but detectable improvement in psoriasis. The adult dose is 5 capsules twice daily; there are no major side-effects but there is a possible interaction with oral anticoagulants.

Epogam capsules (Scotia) contain evening primrose oil providing 40 mg of gamma-linolenic acid. The drug seems able to provide some symptomatic relief for the symptoms of atopic eczema, particularly pruritus. The adult dose is 4—6 capsules daily; no major side-effects have been reported.

Dapsone

For many years monotherapy with the sulphone dapsone was the sole treatment for leprosy. The development of mycobacterial resistance resulted in the adoption of 2- and 3-drug regimens but dapsone is still used in conjunction with rifampicin and clofazimine. Dapsone is the treatment of choice for dermatitis herpetiformis. The exact mechanism of action is uncertain but there appears to be an inhibiting effect on polymorphonuclear leukocyte lysosomal enzymes.

Doses of 50 mg two or three times daily are usual. Safety in pregnancy cannot be guaranteed; Dapsone causes red cell haemolysis and some patients develop a frank haemolytic anaemia. The drug is best avoided in patients who are heterozygous for glucose 6 phosphate dehydrogenase deficiency. Other side-effects include nausea, methaemoglobinaemia, neuropathy and liver damage. Overall however the drug is well tolerated. In combination with pyrimethamine (Maloprim) dapsone is employed for malaria prophylaxis; agranulocytosis is a rare adverse reaction of pyrimethamine. It follows that this preparation is not suitable for the treatment of skin disorders.

4: Other modes of dermatological treatment

Baths

Patients with skin disorders are often given very contradictory advice about the type and frequency of the baths they should take. Unless patients are medically unfit there is never any actual contra-indication to bathing. Baths enable scales, crusts and the residues of old creams to be gently removed. Prolonged contact with water will hydrate the epidermis and some topical preparations, like urea cream, are best applied with the skin in this state. Finally therapeutic agents like oils, tar or antiseptics can be added to the water.

Emollient baths

Emollients act by lubricating the skin and provide a surface film of oil promoting the retention of water. They are reasonably effective substitutes for soap. Emulsifying ointment or aqueous cream can be blended with hot water and added to the bath. Unfortunately residues are left round the bath. Recently water miscible oils have become popular. Oilatum (Stiefel) is a liquid paraffin and acetylated wool alcohols mix. Balneum (Merck) is prepared from soya bean oil and is particularly suitable for lanolin sensitive individuals. Emulsiderm (Dermal) and Alpha Keri (Bristol Myers) are similar products. All should be added to the bath water in accordance with package instructions.

Tar baths

These are not now considered an essential part of the treatment of psoriasis; certainly there is no indication to prescribe anything other than the very acceptable and non-staining proprietary tar bath additives available. Polytar emollient (Stiefel) contains coal tar and oil of cade (birch tar); 20 mls should be added to a bath. Psoriderm Bath Emulsion (Dermal) or Balneum with Tar (Merck) are alternatives.

Antiseptic baths

These are of value in the management of folliculitis, furunculosis and wound infections. In conjunction with other measures topical antiseptics reduce the number of pathogenic bacteria on the skin surface. Savlon hospital concentrate (ICI) contains 1.5% chlorhexidine and 7.5% cetrimide and is supplied in 25 ml sachets. Ster-Zac bath concentrate (Hough, Hoseason) contains 2% triclosan. A 28 ml sachet is added to a 140 litre bath.

Cryotherapy

The destructive effects of low temperatures have been employed by dermatologists, gynaecologists and surgeons for many years. Some employ cryosurgical apparatus where a silver applicator is cooled by allowing a jet of nitrous oxide under pressure to expand rapidly. However most dermatologists use liquid nitrogen as the simplest and most consistent method of destroying benign and malignant skin tumours.

The simplest delivery system for liquid nitrogen is the cotton bud technique. This method is used to treat viral warts. A cotton bud is dipped in liquid nitrogen contained in an all-metal vacuum flask. The bud is then applied vertically onto the lesion. This should be repeated until the wart itself, and 1 mm of the surrounding skin, is frozen. The wart is then allowed to defrost and further lesions selected for treatment. The technique is highly effective for warts on the face and hands and is repeated at intervals of 2−3 weeks until clinical cure. Plantar warts (verrucae) should be pared down before freezing, since keratin insulates, but the technique is less effective on the foot.

It is difficult to treat large lesions adequately and consistently with a cotton bud. A further objection is the possibility that viruses may be transferred from the skin back to the liquid nitrogen flask and remain viable there. A liquid nitrogen spray apparatus e.g. Cryo-Derma (Galderma UK Ltd.) overcomes both these problems. Patches of Bowen's disease, or basal cell carcinomas can be treated satisfactorily with the spray technique. The spray is held 1 cm from the skin surface above the centre of the lesion. After spraying begins a white patch of ice forms which can be enlarged by a rotary motion of the spray tip. The aim is to maintain the lesion, and a 0.5 cm margin of normal skin, frozen for 30 seconds. The area is then allowed to thaw and the process repeated after 5–10 minutes.

If a freezing time of 30 seconds is adopted healing without scarring is usual. The same technique has been adopted to destroy basal cell papillomas, solar keratoses, myxoid cysts and tattoos. If treating malignant tumours the technique should be restricted to those with a clear outer edge. A morphoeic basal cell carcinoma with imprecise margins would not be suitable for treatment in this way.

Treatment of skin disease with ultraviolet radiation

Conventional ultraviolet lamps produce radiation with wavelengths between 290–320 nm (UVB). This form of phototherapy, rather imprecisely termed 'artificial sunlight' has been used for many years to treat psoriasis and acne vulgaris. Photo-chemotherapy (PUVA) is a far more effective, if more complex, treatment for severe psoriasis. Combination treatment with psoralens and long-wave ultra-violet A radiation (320–400 nm) is helpful treatment in perhaps 90% of patients (Table 4.1).

Table 4.1   Criteria for patients being considered for PUVA

Aged over 16 years
Have severe psoriasis (>10% skin involved)
Be physically or socially disabled
Repeated failure to improve with conventional treatment

8-Methoxypsoralen (8-MOP) is a photosensitizer and forms an essential part of the treatment. The drug is taken, with food, 2 hours before UVA exposure. 8-MOP is available in 10 mg tablets; doses between 20 and 60 mg are prescribed on a weight related basis. UVA exposure is provided in a special cabinet lined with UV lamps. The tube output is continuously monitored by a sensor in the cabinet.

The UVA dose is measured in Joules/cm^2. The starting dose is dependent on the individual's skin type or response to natural sunlight (Table 4.2).

Table 4.2 Skin types and response to natural sunlight

Skin type	Response
1	Skin burns and never tans (e.g. red-haired)
2	Skin burns easily; tans with difficulty
3	Skin seldoms burns; tans easily
4	Skin never burns and tans well (e.g. Mediterranean)
5	Permanently brown skin (e.g. Asian)
6	Permanently black skin (e.g. Afro-Caribbean)

UVA doses are increased depending on disease response. Initially patients are treated three times weekly but once a remission is obtained maintenance PUVA sessions can be given less frequently. Protective goggles are worn during treatment since the radiation is potentially damaging to the lens and retina. Patients should avoid sun exposure, and wear polaroid sunglasses, for at least 12 hours after taking a dose of 8-MOP.

There are a number of short-term side-effects of treatment which include pruritus, nausea and erythema. Pigmentation of the skin is invariable, but is usually welcome. Many patients who have received a high total dose of PUVA develop large numbers of pigmented macules on the trunk and limbs.

Psoralens in the presence of UVA causes cross-links between pyrimidine bases in DNA. The combination also has profound immunological effects on the skin. It is not certain which of these actions is of importance in the treatment of psoriasis. PUVA also has a place in the treatment of T-cell lymphoma of the skin (mycosis fungoides) and, possibly, severe atopic eczema.

PUVA is contra-indicated in pregnancy or in patients with a previous history of skin cancer. The incidence of non-melanoma skin tumours reflects the life-time cummulative dose of UV from all sources. It has been suggested that PUVA treatment might increase the risk of developing a tumour of this type by ten fold. Patients with vitiligo would be particularly at risk from skin burning.

5: Management of common skin disorders

Acne vulgaris

Acne vulgaris (Fig. 5.1) usually develops around puberty, with virtually all adolescents being affected to some extent. The age at which it resolves is more variable. Drugs such as androgens and corticosteroids can induce acne at any age. Acne lesions include comedones, inflamed and non-inflamed papules, pustules, nodules, scars and cysts. Areas with a dense population of sebaceous glands (face, back and chest) are principally involved and the severity of the disease is proportional to the sebum production rate.

The successful management of patients with acne requires sympathy and understanding as well as medical knowledge. The disease affects a cosmetically vital area at a psychologically critical period. Reassurance is always important but should not be trivialized by simply telling sufferers that they 'will grow out of it'. Treatment of acne can be based logically on the three main aetiological factors: microbial population, obstruction of the pilo-sebaceous duct, and increased sebum production.

Systemic antibiotics and benzoyl peroxide preparations work by reducing the microbial population of the pilo-sebaceous units, in particular that of *Proprionobacterium acnes*. Any treatment which reduces the adherence of horny plugs that form in follicular ducts is beneficial in acne. Tretinoin (Retin A cream and Gel: Ortho-Cilag) seems to produce this result. Sebum production is promoted by androgens. Some synthetic progesterones, e.g. norgesterol, have an androgenic effect and can exacerbate acne. Cyproterone acetate opposes the peripheral and central effects of androgens. It is available in a combined preparation with the oestrogen ethinyloestradiol (Dianette: Schering). Isotretinoin (Roaccutane, *USA Accutane*: Roche) causes a dramatic reduction in the size of sebaceous glands with a consequential fall in sebum production. It is perhaps the single most effective drug employed in the treatment of acne.

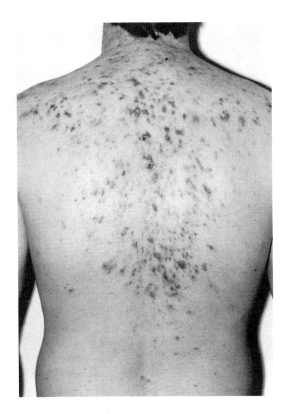

Fig. 5.1 Severe acne vulgaris

Mild acne

A topical agent alone is sufficient. Benzoyl peroxide 2.5% should be prescribed first. A 5% or 10% preparation is substituted if the acne does not improve and if unacceptable irritation is not produced. Tretinoin (Retin A 0.025, 0.05% Cream; 0.025% Gel: Ortho Cilag) is most effective where comedones predominate but can be substituted for benzoyl peroxide in any pattern of acne if this proves ineffective. Both preparations can make the skin dry and erythematous; topical antibiotics can be employed if these side-effects are intolerable.

Moderate acne

Moderately severe acne requires the addition of a systemic antibiotic to a topical preparation. Antibiotics are effective because of their activity against *P. acnes*. The drugs must, however, be used in sufficient dose and duration. Erythromycin or oxytetracycline are both commonly employed. One gram daily for 3–6 months should be prescribed.

Women of reproductive age must be warned about the adverse effects of tetracycline during pregnancy. Systemic preparations are clearly contra-indicated and the safety of the topical preparations cannot be guaranteed. Pregnant patients with acne should be treated with topical benzoyl peroxide; erythromycin is the antibiotic least likely to cause fetal toxicity.

Co-trimoxazole and clindamycin are effective in acne but side-effects such as drug rashes and pseudomembranous colitis have reduced their popularity. The lipid soluble semi-synthetic tetracycline, minocycline (Minocin: Lederle), is very widely prescribed in the UK. It may indeed be worth a trial in patients unresponsive to cheaper drugs used for adequate periods particularly if they have greasy skin.

Concern has been expressed that women with acne using an oral contraceptive may have the effectiveness of their anovulant compromised by an antibiotic. Although such drugs can interfere with the entero-hepatic circulation of oestrogens this does not seem to be a practical problem in acne patients, even those receiving the 30 mcg oestrogen contraceptive pill. However if such patients develop antibiotic associated diarrhoea they should be warned to take additional contraceptive precautions. Female patients unresponsive to, or intolerant of, antibiotic therapy can be treated with Dianette; a course of at least 3 months is necessary.

Severe acne

Severely affected acne patients who have not responded to intensive treatment with conventional agents should be considered for treatment with isotretinoin. At present in the UK this requires hospital referral. Doses of 1.0 mg/Kg are usually given for 3−4 months. Because of its teratogenicity pregnancy should be excluded before treatment is initiated. Effective contraception is necessary during treatment and for 4 weeks after. Side-effects such as cheilitis, nosebleeds, headaches and blepheritis are relatively common but are normally acceptable to individuals whose severe acne is responding.

Minor scarring is common in acne but occasionally this problem can be very severe and unsightly. Early treatment of the active lesions lessens this problem as does explanation to the individual patient that much scarring is the result of self-inflicted excoriation.The injection of acne nodules with 0.1 ml triamcinolone will hasten their resolution and minimize consequential scarring. Remedial camouflage advice is worth offering to all such patients. Although various dietary restrictions have been popular for many years there is no real evidence that they help the average acne sufferer.

Practice points

1 *It is pointless to prescribe short courses of several antibiotics in acne. At least 3−6 months is necessary.*
2 *Avoid tetracycline in children and during pregnancy.*
3 *Be realistic, but optimistic. Refer severe cases and those who have failed to improve with two antibiotics given in adequate doses for appropriate periods.*

Alopecia and scalp disorders

Disorders involving the scalp and hair are the cause of considerable distress. When dealing with affected patients it is helpful to place them in one of the following categories:
• patchy hair loss without scarring (loss of follicles)
• patchy loss with scarring
• diffuse loss
• disease of the scalp without significant hair loss

Alopecia areata is the commonest cause of patchy, non-scarring hair loss in childhood; the disease is by no means rare in adults. Alopecia areata can affect any hairy area although it is usually only noticeable, or worth treating, when it involves the scalp. The scalp in affected sites is smooth and non-inflamed. Short 'exclamation mark' hairs are found at the actively extending margins. The disorder is characterized by an arrest of follicle activity in what is described as a dystrophic anagen phase, followed by a premature telogen. Anagen is the active phase of hair growth and telogen is the resting phase.

An association between alopecia areata and other auto-immune diseases seems unquestionable. If alopecia areata itself is finally proved to be an autoimmune disease it will be unique because no permanent damage is done to the follicle. Hair regrowth is possible after many years of loss. Strangely melanized hairs are more susceptible to damage than 'white' hair.

Attacks of alopecia areata commonly remit spontaneously, but second or third attacks, particularly if associated with atopy or nail pitting, carry a poorer prognosis. If the process advances to involve the entire scalp (alopecia totalis) or the scalp and body hair (alopecia universalis) the chance of improvement is even less.

Regrowth of hair can be achieved with moderate doses of systemic cortico-steroids but relapse occurs almost invariably on drug withdrawal. The side-effects of steroids makes the use of this type of treatment difficult to justify. Topical steroids are widely prescribed although their value is still uncertain. Potent steroid gels and lotions are necessary to obtain any worthwhile effect (e.g. Synalar Gel:ICI; Betnovate Scalp Application: Glaxo). Intralesional triamcinolone can be given through a needleless injector. A tuft of hair may develop at each injection site, although there is a considerable risk of scalp atrophy. This type of treatment may be beneficial in those with persistent but localized hair loss.

Over the last 10 years there have been many trials of new agents in this condition. In some centres the induction of an allergic contact dermatitis (with dinitrochlorobenzene, squaric, acid dibutyl ester or diphencyprone) has been employed as a growth promoting treatment. As yet none of these methods can be said to have achieved an established place in effecting long-term, cosmetically valuable, regrowth.

If acceptable to the patient the provision of wigs can be a very satisfactory solution for the severely affected. In the UK wigs can be supplied biennially by hospital appliance departments if authorised by a dermatologist. Many patients find rapidly progressive hair loss an intensely traumatic experience and will benefit from contact with the appropriate patients' organisation.

In childhood scaly, patchy, alopecia with scarring is likely to be the result of a fungal infection. Rarely a chronic staphylococcal folliculitis (folliculitis decalvans) can produce a scarring pattern of hair loss in adults. Appropriate systemic antibiotics will at least partially control the condition. Scalp involvement by lichen planus and discoid lupus erythematosus (DLE) can cause patchy, scarring alopecia, as can post-radiotherapy damage.

Androgenic alopecia is the commonest cause of non-scarring diffuse hair loss. The process is genetically determined and can affect either sex although the male-pattern alopecia is the more familiar. Typical features are temporal recession of hair and relative sparing of the occipital region. Management is at present both difficult and controversial. Occipital hair transplantation and/or scalp reduction techniques can produce a cosmetic improvement. These surgical procedures are very expensive and require skilled operators if they are to be beneficial. I feel that in general they cannot be recommended. A 2% minoxidil solution is now available in the UK (Regaine: Upjohn) and is being employed topically in the treatment of androgenic alopecia. Approximately one third of patients benefit to some extent but the improvement is not maintained once application is discontinued.

In women thinning of hair over the vertex progresses more slowly and seldom produces complete baldness, although diffuse thinning can eventually be quite marked. The frontal hair line is maintained. The development of this pattern of alopecia in women requires the investigation of hyperandrogenic states such as polycystic ovary syndrome. Anti-androgen treatment may delay progression of the disease.

Diffuse hair loss is common 6–12 weeks after parturition or severe illness. This is termed telogen effluvium. The condition is benign and patients require no treatment, only reassurance that the hair will regrow. There are several other causes of diffuse hair loss:

- thyroid disease
- SLE
- syphilis
- drugs (anti-thyroid agents, cytotoxics, heparin, retinoids)

Hair is often subject to physical trauma. Tight rolling or winding of the hair can result in the so-called 'traction' alopecia in the parietal area. This phenomenon has been described in Sikh children but is occasionally seen in all ethnic groups. When the traction is 'released' it may take many months for even partial improvement to occur. Patients will deliberately pull out their own hair. This type of artefactual hair loss is called trichotillomania and is most common in teenage girls.

Some individuals possess structural or chemical abnormalities of the hair shafts. Shaft defects, such as monilethrix and pili torti, may produce fracture, irregularity, or twisting of the hair.

Not all diseases of the scalp are the cause of significant hair loss. Fine scaling of the scalp is known as pityriasis capitis or dandruff. Other manifestations of seborrhoeic eczema may be present. Regular use of a detergent shampoo will be helpful. Some patients will benefit from shampoos containing selenium sulphide, tar solution or zinc pyrithione. If the scaling is thick 2% salicylic acid in a water soluble base is helpful. More active eczemas of the scalp, like atopic eczema or lichen simplex will require treatment with a topical steroid gel or lotion. Not infrequently 'resistant dandruff' turns out to be scalp psoriasis. In psoriasis the scale is palpable and the involved areas are sharply demarcated from surrounding uninvolved, scalp.

Practice points

1 *Determine the pattern of alopecia before trying to decide on a diagnosis.*

2 *Male pattern alopecia in women, particularly if associated with hirsutism or menstrual irregularity, suggests a disorder of androgen production.*

3 *Even if cure is impossible wigs may still be an effective cosmetic solution to the problem.*

Primary bullous diseases

Blisters or bullae may occur as a feature of several skin disorders such as impetigo, erysipelas, contact dermatitis or insect bites. However the term 'bullous disease' normally refers to a relatively rare group of skin disorders in which vesicle or blister formation is a prominent and primary feature. The disorders present some similarities but can be distinguished on clinical, histological and immunological grounds.

Pemphigus vulgaris is potentially the most serious of these disorders (Fig. 5.2). Superficial fragile blistering and erosions

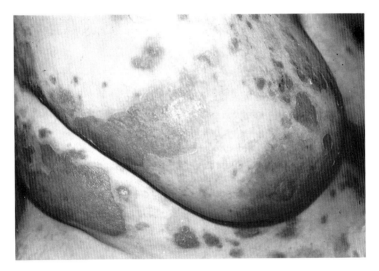

Fig. 5.2 Pemphigus vulgaris producing erosions

are widespread and appear to erupt from normal looking skin. Mucosal surfaces are often severely involved. In pemphigus foliaceous the lesions are erythematous and scaly with oral involvement being unusual. Referral to hospital for biopsy is essential. Histologically acantholysis, or separation of epidermal cells, occurs with antibodies of IgG type being demonstrable in the intracellular spaces. Treatment is with systemic steroids. An initial dose of prednisolone between 60–120 mg daily (1 mg/Kg) is often required to gain control. Once remission is established the dose is gradually reduced to a maintenance level, usually 10–15 mg daily. It is now customary to employ an immunosuppressant such as azathioprine as a 'steroid sparing agent' so that a reduced dose of prednisolone can be prescribed.

Bullous pemphigoid is commoner than pemphigus and generally occurs in the 60–80 age group (Fig. 5.3). Widespread, tense, sub-epidermal blisters form, often on an urticarial or erythematous base. Oral involvement in pemphigoid is rare. Some patients may have generalized itching for months before the classical rash occurs; others develop a rash of the hands and feet which closely resembles a haemorrhagic pompholyx.

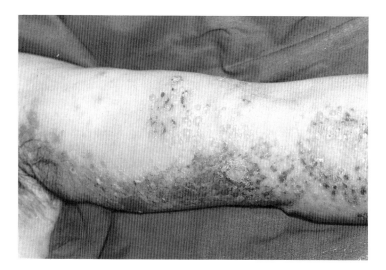

Fig. 5.3 Bullous pemphigoid; commoner than pemphigus

On skin biopsy bands of IgG and complement can usually be demonstrated at the dermo-epidermal junction. Bullous pemphigoid is managed in a similar way to pemphigus although a starting dose of prednisolone in the 30–40 mg (0.5 mg/Kg) range is often sufficient and the use of a steroid sparing agent is not always required. A rarer variant of pemphigoid (benign mucous membrane pemphigoid) is usually confined to the eyes and mouth.

Dermatitis herpetiformis (DH) produces intensely itchy vesicles and urticarial papules which appear on the shoulder, elbows, arms, sacrum and knees. DH is slightly commoner in males than females and usually presents in the 15–40 age group. Clinical diagnosis is often difficult and delayed. Histologically splitting is seen at the tips of the dermal papillae, and granular deposition of IgA occurs at the dermo-epidermal junction, even in uninvolved skin. Dapsone is a very effective treatment for this disease. The pruritus may disappear within a day or two of commencing the drug and indeed the response to dapsone is virtually a diagnostic test. The dose required to control DH is usually within 50–150 mg per day. Sulphapyridine (500 mg twice daily) is an alternative but less effective drug usually employed if dapsone causes unacceptable haemolysis. Once initiated therapy is required for years, if not life.

Patients with DH have a gluten-sensitive enteropathy although only a minority have coeliac disease symptoms. It is generally agreed that a gluten free diet greatly improves DH with the requirement for dapsone being substantially reduced. Unfortunately it is arduous to stick to a diet of this type and absolute avoidance indefinitely appears to be necessary. The rash usually takes 6 months to improve and naturally foods containing wheat, barley and rye flour in any form must not be consumed.

Practice points

1 *Try to decide if blistering is primary or secondary.*
2 *Although described as bullous diseases intact blisters may not be prominent in DH and pemphigus.*

3 *Histology and immunohistology are essential in the evaluation of a primary bullous disorder and this requires hospital referral.*

Dermatitis artefacta and psychogenic skin disease

Simulated skin disease is by no means uncommon and can be most difficult to recognize. It is widely accepted that patients are more likely to approach their doctors with physical symptoms, rather than mention psychological diffulties at the beginning of a consultation. This phenomenon has recently been described as 'somatization'. Sadly patients who have adopted this form of defence against unacceptable feelings or emotions may have lengthy, and entirely unsatisfactory, careers as dermatological out-patients.

Dermatitis artefacta (DA)

DA naturally affects those sites which are accessible (Fig. 5.4). Patients often give a rather unconvincing or 'hollow' history.

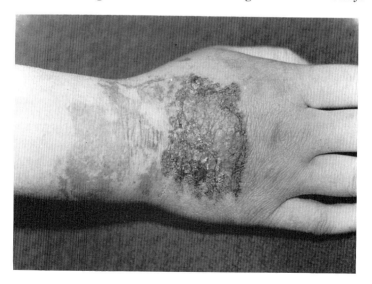

Fig. 5.4 Dermatitis artefacta; geometrical in shape

The lesions are often geometrical in shape and may show superficial necrosis or ulceration. They are difficult to explain in terms of common skin disorders and will heal naturally if the area can be occluded. A few of the patients are frankly psychotic but the vast majority have no gross psychopathology. In many individuals it is difficult to see what benefit results from the simulation and DA seldom, if ever, represents simple malingering for some clearly definable purpose. Adults with DA are notoriously reluctant to accept psychiatric help but I feel that expert assessment is necessary with children. The advice of a child psychiatrist or child and family unit should be sought.

Acne excoriée

Acne excoriée is a disease normally seen in young women. Multiple excoriations are seen over the face and shoulders sometimes, but not always, associated with mild acne. Treatment with antibiotics and antihistamines may be of some marginal benefit. Many patients with this disorder accept that they scratch or pick themselves unreasonably but this insight does not always lead to improvement.

Delusional parasitosis

This disorder, previously known as parasitophobia, entails the unshakeable belief by a patient that his or her skin is infested with insects. Infrequently the delusion is caused by an organic brain syndrome. For such an apparently bizarre phenomenon the delusion can be remarkably stereotyped. Most patients proffer a small envelope containing skin fragments with which to support their diagnosis. This, to quote W.S. Gilbert, is 'merely corroborative detail intended to give artistic verisimilitude to an otherwise bald and unconvincing narrative'. Maintaining a rapport with the deluded victims can be difficult; it seems essential not to confront them with the reality that no insects exist. Once again patients resist psychiatric referral although the neuroleptic drug pimozide (Orap: Janssen) 4–10 mg daily can at least partially control the syndrome in many patients.

Disorders of body-image

Patients with this condition have an excessive, and often obsessive, preoccupation with the shape of their nose, breasts or their facial hair or non-existent baldness. If anything these patients are even more difficult to deal with than the previous groups. The very nature of the disorder means that a suggested psychiatric referral is almost certain to be rejected. It is difficult to support such patients without colluding in their delusion, yet their distress is very real. Some may accept antidepressants or long-term supportive psychotherapy, and a very few may benefit.

TATTOOS, EAR-PIERCING AND DESIRED ARTEFACTS

Tattoos are consciously produced artefacts which may be of cultural, social or purely aesthetic significance (Fig. 5.5). In the UK the establishments of professional tattooists must be inspected by, and registered with, the local authority. It is not legal for professionals to tattoo minors under 18 years although

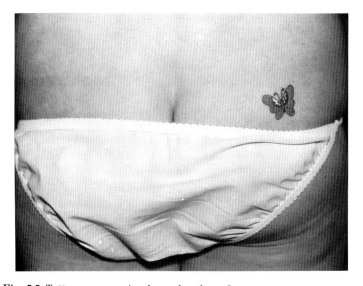

Fig. 5.5 Tattoos are consciously produced artefacts

there are plenty of amateurs at work in schools and corrective institutions (Table 5.1).

Table 5.1   Hazard of tattoos

Allergy to the pigments employed
Sarcoidal reactions
Keloid scarring
Transmission of syphilis and hepatitis

Naturally many of those tattooed eventually wish to have their embellishments removed. Unless the design is small enough to be treated by direct excision and closure this will present difficulties. Abrasion with salt, cryotherapy and laser-shave have all been employed with varying degrees of success.

Ear-piercing, even multiple ear-piercing, is a socially acceptable artefact. Nose-piercing in the UK is traditional in females from the Asian community and is just about on the right side of respectability in the white community. Mercifully nipple and labial-piercing have not as yet obtained widespread acceptance. Ear-piercing commonly results in infection and keloid formation, and may be the cause of the high incidence of nickel sensitivity in women.

Various ethnic medical traditions practice counter-irritation techniques such as cupping, blistering and coin rolling which can produce initially puzzling skin signs.

Practice points

1 *Like diamonds tattoos are, almost always, forever.*
2 *Suspect dermatitis artefacta if a skin lesion does not conform to any familiar disorder and inexplicably fails to heal.*
3 *An ostensibly physical problem, such as alopecia or hyper-trichosis, which is completely undetectable will not be organic in origin.*

Drug eruptions

Any drug can cause any rash at any time but the frequency and variety of drug eruptions seen reflects the pattern of contemporary prescribing. Drugs can cause damage in many ways. The dermal atrophy associated with steroids and the cheilitis caused by isotretinoin are inevitable pharmacological side-effects. Drug hypersensitivity implies the operation of the immune system; a number of clinical patterns can be produced in this way including urticaria, vasculitis and cell-mediated contact dermatitis. An idiosyncratic reaction is a highly abnormal effect of a drug which does not involve the immune system; toxic epidermal necrolysis is an example.

When taking a drug history it is important to question the patient about over-the-counter medication such as laxatives and analgesics.

Acneiform

Acne-like rashes, rather monomorphic in type, are associated with systemic steroids, androgens, isoniazid and iodides.

Exanthematic

The exanthematic or morbilliform rash is the most common pattern of all. A good example is the 'ampicillin' eruption (Fig. 5.6). The mechanism is thought to be allergic in type although the ampicillin rash seen during infectious mononucleosis is probably an exception to this. The ampicillin rash usually develops 7–10 days after first exposure. Second exposures can produce the rash within hours. Among the many drugs that produce this pattern are other penicillins, sulphonamides, allopurinol, barbiturates, phenytoin, carbamazepine, analgesics, penicillamine, and gold.

Fixed drug eruption

This extra-ordinary rash recurs at exactly the same sites on each exposure to the drug. Lesions are often oval or circular and in white skin have a unique brownish-red colour. Healing with pigmentation is usual. Since phenolphthalein causes this problem it is important to enquire about laxatives. Other drugs involved are quinine, sulphonamides, chlordiazepoxide, and analgesics. Fixed eruptions caused by tetracycline may pulsate.

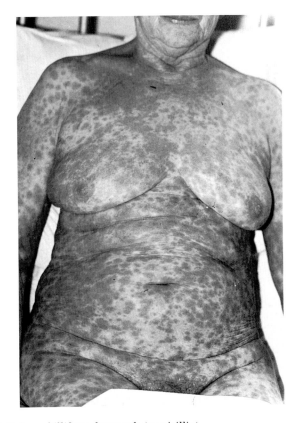

Fig. 5.6 A morbilliform drug rash (ampicillin)

Lichenoid

Lichenoid reactions do not exactly resemble lichen planus. Either the morphology of individual lesions, or their distribution, differs from the classical dermatosis. Methyldopa, thiazides, chloroquine, quinine and gold are all associated with lichenoid rashes.

Pigmentation

Pigmentation develops on the skins of patients treated long-term with phenothiazines. Amiodarone produces pigmentation unrelated to photo-sensitivity. Busulphan and phenytoin are also known to be associated with this change. Minocycline therapy may result in a bluish pigmentation of acne scars and patches of similar colour change in the skin. Once the drug is stopped the colour fades over several months.

Toxic epidermal necrolysis (TEN)

This rare and most dangerous drug reaction has a mortality rate of 25–50%. Large areas of the skin becomes red and swollen. The epidermis separates in large sheets. Mouth and gastro-intestinal involvement is usual. Virtually all drugs have occasionally been linked with TEN but evidence is often only circumstantial. The link is reasonably assured with sulphonamides, barbiturates, carbamazepine, allopurinol, analgesics, and the penicillins.

Other dangerous drug rashes include erythroderma and Stevens-Johnson syndrome (severe erythema multiforme). Sulphonamides, gold, phenylbutazone and phenytoin have been linked with reactions of this type.

Urticarial

Drugs can produce urticaria in two ways. Aspirin can cause the release of vaso-active amines by a direct effect on mast cells. Other drugs may work through an immunological effect. Either way the agents involved include morphine, penicillin, aspirin, codeine, and radio-contrasts.

Practice points

1 *Always enquire about previous drug allergy before prescribing.*
2 *A drug rash is more likely to be the result of a recently prescribed drug.*
3 *Remember the drug may have been stopped before the rash appears.*

Eczema, atopic

The management of atopic eczema dominates the practice of paediatric dermatology. Although the overall tendency is improvement with age 50% of patients discover that their problem persists into adult life (Fig. 5.7 and 5.8). An itchy rash characteristically begins on the face and napkin area at 3–6 months Later the problem localises to the wrists, feet, buttocks and flexures. Some adults lose their eczema at all sites except the hands. The disease often occurs in association with asthma or hayfever, and commonly shows familial aggregation.

Atopic skin is generally dry and exhibits white dermographism. Active eczema is scaly, erythematous and excoriated. Chronic eczematous patches frequently show thickening with prominence of the skin creases (lichenification). Patients with atopic eczema are susceptible to many skin infections. They may contract severe herpes simplex (Kaposi's varicelliform eruption), warts or molluscum contagiosum. Secondary bacterial infection (usually with *Staphylococcus aureus*) results in weeping and crusting with increased itch and soreness.

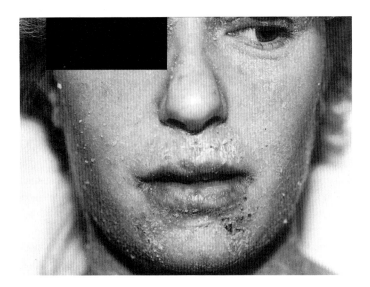

Fig. 5.7 Atopic eczema of the face

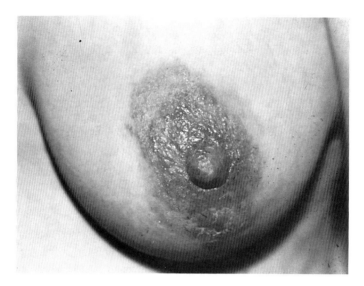

Fig. 5.8 Primary nipple eczema; not Paget's disease

Investigation of the eczema is not usually very rewarding. A skin swab may make planning antibiotic therapy more logical. The serum IgE level will usually be raised, and most atopic individuals will have multiple positive prick tests to common ingestants and inhalents (e.g. egg, milk, grass pollen, cat epithelium and house-dust mite).

Before treatment commences it must be clearly explained that regular therapy is essential, and that the eczema can be greatly improved but not cured. It is disturbing to see patients present with a large carrier bag full of half-empty tubes of topical steroids who have never been given a diagnosis nor had their treatment properly planned. Advisory leaflets like those produced by the National Eczema Society have a valuable educative function and are available in English and several Asian languages. If the patient is of school age I would recommend keeping the school informed particularly since treatment with antihistamines may lead to deterioration in classroom performance.

It is important, particularly in children, to obtain the maximum possible benefits from the regular use of emollients e.g.

Aqueous Cream, Diprobase, Unguentum Merk or E45 cream. Irritants, such as wool worn next to the skin and soap, should be avoided. Aqueous cream or bath emollients such as Oilatum (Stiefel) and Balneum (Merck) should be used as soap substitutes. The daily application of a topical steroid can be very helpful. Only hydrocortisone preparations are safe enough to be used regularly on babies and toddlers. Hydrocortisone 1% cream or ointment are cheap and safe, with the ointment being the more effective base. Vioform-Hydrocortisone (Ciba) is useful in the presence of secondary infection. Dry skin will benefit from 10% Urea Cream with (Alphaderm; Calmurid-HC) or without (Aquadrate; Calmurid) hydrocortisone. Older children and adults may use low potency fluorinated topical steroids such as Eumovate or Haelan ointments. Even with such relatively weak preparations use on the face and flexures should be minimized.

Potent preparation (e.g. Betnovate; Synalar) should be used as brief courses in severely affected adults. If you elect to use these preparations try the manufacturer's diluted formulations first (e.g. Betnovate RD; Synalar 1/4 or 1/10). Coal tar pastes and ointments can be helpful for dry, thick lichenified plaques of eczema and can be applied at night under Tubegauz or Stockinette bandages. Coal tar derivatives are messy but safe. Lichenification can occur in all ethnic groups but is particularly common, and troublesome, in Afro-Caribbean children.

Systemic treatment is usually considered for severe atopic eczema in relapse. Virtually all such patients will have their skin colonized by *Staph. aureus* and an appropriate antibiotic like erythromycin or flucloxacillin will be helpful. Sedative antihistamines reduce night time itching. Trimeprazine syrup is safe and widely used. Older children are quite tolerant of its effects and 15–30 mg doses may be required. Hydroxyzine syrup 10–20 mg is an alternative.

Despite the great interest presently shown in the subject I have found the use of elimination diets disappointing. A few infants do seem to improve with egg, dairy product and azo-dye free diets but I do not recommend these unless conventional treatment has failed. Such regimes can result in malnutrition and should not be provided without skilled dietetic help. Patients should be forbidden to give unpasteurized goat's milk to small children. Patients with atopic eczema have been reported to have lower than normal levels of gamma-linolenic acid and its metabolites. Because of this dietary supplements in the form of evening primrose oil (Epogam: Scotia) have recently become popular. Adults will need 4–6 capsules twice daily and response may be delayed for 2–3 months. It is too early to say if this form of treatment will obtain a recognized place in the management of eczema.

Treatment with ultraviolet light, (UVB) phototherapy will help some individuals. Housedust mite avoidance may be of value. Affected patients should have their pillows and matresses covered in plastic sheeting and have their bedrooms vacuumed and damp-dusted twice weekly. They should not lounge around on carpets.

The value of systemic corticosteroids in eczema is debateable. There use should be restricted to patients who are seriously disabled by their disease, and in whom all other forms of treatment have failed. It is doubtful if children ever fulfil these criteria and even in adults the employment of short courses of prednisolone or ACTH are rarely needed.

Practical points

1 *A tube of a potent topical steroid is no solution to infantile eczema.*
2 *Make sure that the benefits of safe treatments like emollients are fully exploited.*
3 *Atopic children benefit from a therapeutic partnership which may include the family doctor, the dermatologist, the school teacher, the dietician and themselves.*

Eczema, other constitutional patterns

The two terms 'eczema' and 'dermatitis' are confusingly applied to the same inflammatory pattern of skin response. Some dermatologists use the words as synonyms, others restrict 'eczema' to constitutional or endogenous patterns and use 'dermatitis' when external or exogenous factors are of prime importance.

Seborrhoeic eczema

Seborrhoeic eczema is common in sites of high sebaceous gland density although there is no evidence that any abnormality in sebum is directly responsible for its development. There are a variety of clinical patterns. Diffuse scaling of the scalp is almost invariable and blepheritis is common. Redness and greasy scaling are prominent on the eyebrows, cheeks and naso-labial folds. A similar rash may involve the presternal area. In the flexures, seborrhoeic eczema presents as an intertrigo with soreness, erythema and scaling. A crusted fissure often develops in the retro-auricular area.

This pattern of constitutional eczema is very steroid sensitive. The regular use of hydrocortisone 1% will normally control the problem although relapses are frequent. For years the role of the yeast *Pityrosporum orbiculare* in the production of seborrhoeic eczema has been discussed. Some patients seem to respond better to an imidazole/hydrocortisone mixture, like Canesten-HC (Bayer) than to the steroid alone. Ketoconazole shampoo (Janssen) has recently been introduced for control of seborrhoeic dermatitis of the scalp. Shampoos containing tar or selenium sulphide are also moderately effective in this disorder.

Pompholyx

This condition is a resistant palmo-plantar eczema (Fig. 5.9). It is frequently disabling with patients developing large blisters on the palms and soles. In more chronic cases innumerable vesicles, resembling tapioca grains, are seen. Severe acute vesicular pompholyx is unresponsive to topical steroid treatment. Potassium permanganate soaks combined with antibiotics and systemic steroids are usually required. As the activity of the attack subsides the systemic steroids can be discontinued and a potent topical preparation substituted.

The use of superficial X-ray therapy to treat benign disorders is declining but this is one condition which does seem to respond well to radiation. Whatever treatment is employed relapses must be anticipated.

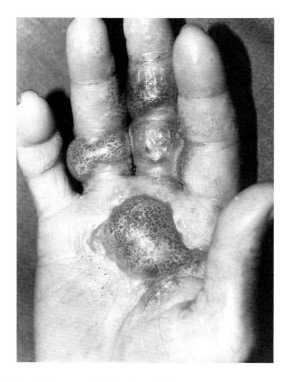

Fig. 5.9 Pompholyx; resistant palmo-plantar eczema

Lichen simplex chronicus

This condition is a variety of long-standing, localized, eczema in which thickening of the epidermis with prominent skin creases (lichenification) predominates. The lesions are often solitary with the lower legs, forearms, occipital area and ano-genital region commonly involved. Occlusive dressing with tar impregnated bandages is valuable if the anatomy of the affected site permits. Otherwise the use of coal tar ointment, or a steroid-salicylic acid ointment (Diprosalic: Kirkby Warwick) may be helpful. Resistant areas of lichen simplex may require treatment with a high potency steroid ointment or superficial X-ray therapy. Relapses are common.

Discoid eczema

Discoid or nummular eczema usually affects the middle-aged or elderly but a similar pattern is seen in young atopics. Scaling, itchy, erythematous discs develop particularly on the arms or legs. Discoid eczema responds to topical steroid treatment although a potent preparation in an ointment base is normally required.

Erythroderma

Erythrodermic patients are red, and often scaly, all over (see Plate 1). This phenomenon was previously described as exfoliative 'dermatitis' but although an eczematous reaction is a common cause of erythroderma it is not invariable (Table 5.2).

Table 5.2   Causes of erythroderma

Eczema
Psoriasis
Lymphoma and leukaemia
Drug reactions
Ichthyosis and related disorders
Idiopathic

Erythrodermic patients suffer substantial fluid and protein loss through their skin. Temperature regulation is difficult and circulatory problems are common, particularly in the elderly. Erythroderma is a dermatological emergency. Patients should be nursed in a warm room and given adequate fluid, electrolyte and protein replacement. Most will require systemic steroids in addition to specific treatment for the underlying condition.

Contact dermatitis

Allergic contact dermatitis is a T-lymphocyte mediated delayed hypersensitivity. The problem is often easy to recognize, and there is a confirmatory investigation, the patch test. Chemicals

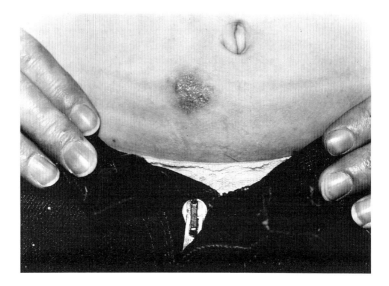

Fig. 5.10 Contact dermatitis to nickel (zip fastener)

vary in their capacity to act as sensitizers. Some, such as dinitrochlorobenzene, will sensitize all immunologically normal subjects. There may be a differential sex incidence; nickel dermatitis is much commoner in women than men (Fig. 5.10).

The chemicals concerned may sensitize in their own right or act as haptens in association with epidermal protein. It seems likely that the resulting complex is phagocytosed by epidermal Langerhans' cells and then transferred by these cells to regional lymph nodes. Here a population of modified T-lymphocytes are produced. After 5–10 days the individual is said to be sensitized and further exposure to the chemical concerned will result in a contact dermatitis within 24–48 hours.

In a patch test the suspected substance, or more usually a battery of likely substances, is suspended in a diluent (usually water or soft paraffin) in an appropriate concentration. Small quantities are then applied to the skin of the back under an occlusive patch and left undisturbed for 48 hours. On removal of the patch erythema and vesiculation indicate a positive

Table 5.3 Common causes of contact dermatitis

Nickel	Cheap jewellery; clothing clips; coins
Chromium	Cement; plaster; dye mordant
Colophony	Sticking plaster; rosin; solder flux
Epoxy resin	Adhesives and plastics
Rubber additives	Gloves; tyres; barrier contraceptives
Neomycin	⎫
Parabens	⎪
Chlorocresol	⎬ Medicaments and cosmetics
Lanolin	⎪
Local anaethetics	⎭
Primin	*Primula obconica* plant dermatitis
Fragrances	Perfumes; cosmetics
p-phenylene diamine	Permanent hair dye

reaction. Not infrequently positive reactions continue to develop for a further 48 hours or even longer and it is usual to 'read' patch tests at 48 and 96 hours.

In many circumstances, and certainly within an industrial setting, irritant dermatitis is more common than allergic contact dermatitis. The use of industrial irritants in patch tests, without consideration of appropriate pre-dilution, may lead to spurious irritant false positives which are at best irrelevant and at worst completely misleading.

Hand eczema, particularly the 'housewives dermatitis' type, is frequently an irritant problem (Table 5.4). Involvement of the thin skin on the back of the hand is common whereas constitutional eczema (pompholyx) usually affects the palm. The changes are most obvious on the patient's dominant hand. Eczema under a wedding ring, which is common in this situation, represents the result of retained irritant detergent residues, not a gold allergy!

Table 5.4 Common irritants

Solvents, degreasing agents
Acids, alkalis
Soaps, detergents
Cutting and coolant oils
Vegetable juices

After diseases of the chest dermatitis must represent the largest group of occupational disorders. Such problems are commonly seen in hairdressers, chemical process workers, engineers, nurses and in the catering and construction trades. The development of an occupational dermatitis can profoundly affect the patient's prospects of employment and may result in litigation. I would not recommend general practitioners to advise on such problems without specialist guidance.

Patients with a contact dermatitis must avoid the material to which they are allergic. It can be difficult to track down all the sources of exposure. Patient information sheets are very helpful. A topical steroid would be appropriate local treatment but is unlikely to be successful alone if exposure continues. Some patterns of contact dermatitis respond to social engineering. The replacement of stockings by tights (pantyhose) resulted in the virtual disappearance of nickel 'suspender dermatitis'. The incidence of chromium related cement dermatitis in Scandinavia has been greatly reduced by the addition of 1% ferrous sulphate to the cement which apparently lowers the amount of soluble chromate present.

Practice points

1 *There is no completely reliable clinical way of distinguishing a constitutional eczema from a contact dermatitis.*

2 *Irritant contact dermatitis is commoner than allergic contact dermatitis.*

3 *Patients whose employment is put at risk by a dermatitis should be referred to a dermatologist.*

Erythema multiforme and related disorders

Erythema multiforme

Erythema multiforme (EM) is a cutaneous reaction pattern associated with several antecedents:
- viral infection (e.g. herpes simplex)
- *Mycoplasma pneumoniae* infection
- drugs (e.g. phenytoin, sulphonamides)

- leukaemia
- post radiotherapy

The rash affects the hands, forearms, knees and feet most profusely. Individually the lesions consist of erythematous macules with a central bluish or bullous area; this appearance has been likened to a 'target'. Mucosal involvement is common. Severe involvement of the mouth, eyes and genitalia associated with a more generalized rash is known as Stevens–Johnson syndrome.

If a cause for EM is discovered then this should, if possible, be treated. It is doubtful if any treatment will shorten an attack once this is initiated. Tetracycline mouth wash may help oral ulceration. The value of systemic steroids is uncertain although these drugs are frequently used in Stevens–Johnson syndrome. Herpes simplex infection may be associated with up to 50% of cases of EM. The problem typically occurs in older children and young adults with the EM arising 7–10 days after the virus infection. Prophylactic oral acyclovir is the only reliable way of preventing these episodes.

Toxic erythema

'Toxic' erythema is a morbilliform rash. The lesions are often urticated and may be generalized or localized to the limbs. Toxic erythema is frequently a drug eruption and may be caused by ampicillin, phenothiazines or thiazides. The rash can also be post-streptococcal or follow viral infections. Many patients have no obvious antecedent cause but the problem is usually self-limiting. Systemic antihistamines or topical steroids may provide symptomatic relief.

Sweet's syndrome

Sweet's syndrome consists of a striking erythematous rash often associated with constitutional symptoms such as fever and arthralgia. It is rare but quite easily recognizable and probably under-reported. The majority, perhaps 80%, of patients with Sweet's syndrome are female, usually between the ages of 30–60.

Classically the syndrome is a combinatioin of fever, a poly-morphonuclear leucocytosis in the peripheral blood and a rash consisting of asymmetrical dusky erythematous nodules which are more usually found on the head, neck and limbs than on the trunk. The lesions are tender, enlarge slowly, and often coalesce. Their appearance has been graphically likened to the relief model of a mountain range. Following corticosteroid therapy the fever rapidly abates. There is complete resolution of the rash without scarring, although residual pigmentation can be prominent.

Hidradenitis suppurativa (apocrine acne)

Those affected by this unpleasant and painful disease develop recurrent 'boils' or pustules. The disease occurs after puberty and seems definitely to be androgen related. It is commoner in women than men and there may be a family history. Hidra-denitis is not a simple pyogenic infection but rather a chronic inflammatory and scarring process affecting apocrine sweat glands, or at least areas containing these glands, such as the axillary, submammary, inguinal, and perianal regions (Fig. 5.11). Inflammation in apocrine sweat glands spreads out into the subcutaneous tissue and severely affected individuals ex-hibit abscesses, sinus tracts and deep scars.

The role of bacterial infection in this disease is controversial but it seems reasonable to treat any organism isolated with an appropriate antibiotic and to employ topical antiseptics, such as Hibiscrub. The use of long-term antibiotics, such as tetra-cycline, minocycline or clindamycin, in 'anti-acne' regimes for 6 months can sometimes be helpful.

Some female patients find that attacks of hidradenitis are precipitated by use of the oral contraceptive pill; for these an alternative form of contraception would be desirable. Since the disease is almost certainly androgen related cyproterone ace-tate may be helpful in the treatment of female patients in regimes like those mentioned in the sections on hirsutism and acne. Isotretinoin is sometimes prescribed under hospital supervision but is not as beneficial in hidradenitis as it is in acne.

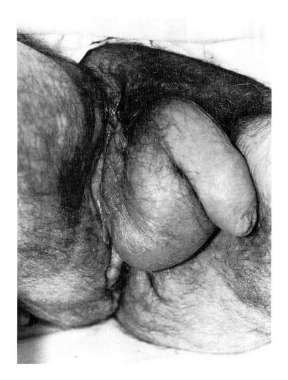

Fig. 5.11 Severe ano-genital hidradenitis suppurativa

Total surgical excision of affected areas is at present the most reliable method of dealing with this disease and must be considered the treatment of choice for severely affected patients. All the apocrine gland bearing skin and subcutaneous tissue must be excised from an affected area which is then allowed to heal by granulation or is covered with a split skin graft.

Practice points

1 *Do not assume that an axillary abscess is necessarily staphylococcal.*
2 *Give all patients a trial on long-term antibiotics.*
3 *Most severely affected patients will benefit from surgery.*

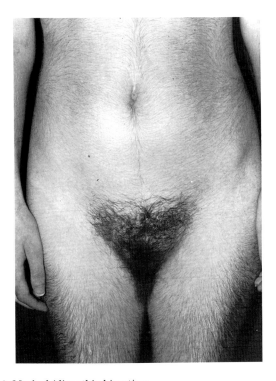

Fig. 5.12 Marked idiopathic hirsutism

Hirsutism and hypertrichosis

Coarse 'terminal' hair develops from fine 'vellus' hair under androgenic stimulation (Fig. 5.12). Hirsutism is the development of male pattern secondary sexual hair by a female (Table 5.5). Localized development of unwanted terminal hair, in either sex, is more correctly described as hypertrichosis. At least 95% women who develop hirsutism are endocrinologically normal. Rarely the symptom is one manifestation of a true virilization syndrome which includes increased muscle bulk, temporal recession of the scalp hair, acne or seborrhoea, breast shrinkage, menstrual disturbance and cliteromegaly.

Full androgen investigation must be performed if the hirsutism is progressive, if menstrual periods are irregular or if

Table 5.5 Disorders associated with hirsutism

Drugs administration, e.g. steroids, androgens
Polycystic ovary syndrome (Stein–Leventhal)
Cushing's syndrome
Androgen secreting tumours (adrenal or ovarian)
Adreno-genital syndrome

other features of virilization are present. In practice those who are ostensibly healthy, whose hirsutism began around puberty, who are on no drugs, and who have a regular menstrual cycle and normal physical examination are extremely unlikely to have a definable and treatable cause for their problem and are said to have idiopathic hirsutism. Mild degrees of hirsutism are particularly common in Asian girls.

The very real distress and embarrassment suffered by hirsute women arises from the irrational perception in western society that the perfect female is slim, tall and has unblemished, hairless, skin.

Physical and chemical methods of hair removal

These are an essential part of all therapeutic regimes and for many patients are the only forms of treatment offered. Shaving is simple and effective. Because of its association with masculinity most women are reluctant to use razors to remove facial hair, but not hair on the body or limbs. Waxing is also an effective technique offered by most beauty therapists. The epilation creams available commercially are based on powerful reducing agents that split the disulphide bonds in keratin with resulting disruption of the hair. Calcium thioglycollate is a common example of such an agent. In the long-run regular use of epilation creams is expensive, and some patients find them too irritating to use on the face. Electrolysis is the only permanently effective method of hair removal. It is most suitable for localized hairy areas but requires a skilled operator, is time-consuming and expensive. It is not widely available within the NHS.

Drugs

The regular use of the oral contraceptive Dianette may be beneficial because it contains the anti-androgen cyproterone acetate. (CPA) antagonises the central and peripheral effects of androgens. Mild idiopathic hirsutism can show improvement within 3–6 months of treatment but relapse occurs once the drug is discontinued. Minor side-effects, like breast tenderness, are relatively common. More severely affected patients can be given additional CPA during 10 days of the cycle.

Practice points

1 *Begin treatment by assuring the patient of her normality.*
2 *Get the maximum possible benefit from physical removal techniques.*

Hyperhidrosis and sweating disorders

Excessive local sweating is an embarrassing problem which normally develops at puberty and, fortunately, usually remits spontaneously in the late twenties. Axillary sweating is of variable extent and severity. If shaving and proprietary antiperspirants are insufficient then a saturated alcoholic solution of aluminium chloride hexahydrate should then be applied. Three preparations are available Anhydrol Forte (Dermal), Hyperdrol (BritCair) and Driclor (Stiefel).

Initially the procedure should be performed on two successive nights. Thereafter one or two applications weekly should be sufficient. Contact with sweat may result in the formation of irritant hydrochloric acid by hydrolysis. It is thus essential that the preparation is applied to a dry, non-sweating, axilla last thing at night and washed off in the morning; the treatment should not be performed on the same day that the axillae are shaved. Hydrocortisone cream 1% may help to offset unavoidable irritation. If medical treatment fails and the problem is both severe and disturbing to the patient then referral for surgical excision of the axillary skin would be justified.

Hyperhidrosis of the soles can be complicated by the development of pitted keratolysis (keratolysis plantare sulcatum). Maceration, shallow pits and superficial erosions are visible in the horny layer of the skin of the soles and toes. There may be obvious signs of secondary infection and an offensive odour is invariable. It is presumed that a micro-organism, possibly a corynaebacterium, invades keratin softened by excessive sweating, although the exact cause of the disorder is still the subject of debate. Combination treatment with an astringent (like potassium permanganate 0.01%) and an antimicrobial (such as Fucidin or miconazole cream) is usually helpful.

Simple hyperhidrosis of the feet and fingers can be troublesome enough. Perspiration may drip off the fingers constantly which is very inconvenient indeed if it affects writing, playing a musical instrument or work. A saturated solution of aluminium chloride can be applied to the hands or feet although the treatment is less successful than in the axillae. If topical treatment fails most physiotherapy departments can arrange iontophoresis with tap-water or the atropine-like drug glycopyrronium (Robinul: Robins). If all else fails and the patient is sufficiently disabled then sympathectomy can be considered. This is by no means a trivial procedure and the hyperhidrosis may eventually return.

Generalized hyperhidrosis is a rare but intractable problem. Occasionally thyrotoxicosis or an underlying lymphoma may be discovered. Generalized sweating has also been associated with a variety of neurological problems. Some patients can tolerate propantheline bromide (Pro-Banthine: Gold Cross) in doses of up to 90 mg daily which may be beneficial.

Miliaria

Miliaria crystallina consists of small vesicles at the sweat duct openings that have the appearance of dry jelly. The disorder is asymptomatic and requires no treatment. It may complicate severe sunburn and febrile illnesses. Miliaria rubra is the result of sweat gland occlusion at a deeper level. An erythematous and vesicular rash results. In the UK miliaria rubra usually afflicts overclothed babies during the summer months.

Once the child is clothed more sensibly the problem settles within a few days.

Practice point

Excessive sweating is quite a common complaint. Only refer the most severely affected. These patients can be recognized by the visible sweat droplets on the skin and a history of saturated, rotting, clothing.

Ichthyosis and related disorders

The ichthyoses are disorders of keratinization which produce the familiar dry and scaly skin. The majority of patients seen have the familial types although rare acquired forms have been described in association with malabsorption and lymphoma.

There are a number of patterns of inheritance but the commonest is an autosomal dominant type (ichthyosis vulgaris). This is frequently associated with atopic eczema. The skin in this condition is dry and rough although the flexures are spared. The condition is usually more trouble in the winter than in the summer. The recessive X-linked pattern of ichthyosis is the result of a metabolic defect. The enzyme steroid sulphatase is deficient in the skin, placenta and other tissues. Severe and generalized recessive types such as lamellar ichthyosis and bullous ichthyosiform erythroderma are very rare. Naturally they are commoner if there is a history of parental consanguinity and affected children may present at birth as 'collodion babies'.

Many patients find simple emollients helpful. E45 cream, Unguentum Merck and Ultrabase are widely used. Emulsifying ointment, Oilatum (Stiefel) or Balneum (Merck) can be added to the bath.

A 10% urea cream is very helpful in hyperkeratotic states. Examples are Calmurid (Pharmacia) and Aquadrate (Eaton). These should be applied in a thick layer after bathing. The cream should be left on the skin for a few minutes then rubbed in and the excess removed. A viscous lotion containing lactic acid and sodium pyrrolidone (Lacticare: Stiefel) is also worth trying.

Until recently there was no systemic treatment helpful in the management of ichthyosis. The new retinoid, etretinate (Tigason: Roche), can be beneficial is some severe cases but because of its side-effects it is a far from ideal therapeutic agent.

Keratosis pilaris

Keratosis pilaris (KP) is a spiky hyperkeratosis affecting the hair follicle orifices. KP may accompany ichthyosis or atopic eczema but can also be an isolated finding; there is often a family history. The complaint is usually most obvious over the outer aspects of the upper arms although involvement of the thighs is also common. KP presents in childhood or adolescence and tends to improve with time and sunlight. Urea cream 10% (Calmurid: Pharmacia) or 2% salicylic acid ointment reduces the hyperkeratosis.

Practice points

1 *All patients with ichthyosis should see a dermatologist at least once for a complete diagnosis to be made. This may require a skin biopsy.*
2 *Parents of children with ichthyosis should receive genetic counselling.*

Bacterial infections

Pyogenic infections

Staphylococci and streptococci are the commonest causes of bacterial skin infections. Streptococci (usually of Lancefield Group A) cause acute and recurrent erysipelas. *Staphylococcus aureus* produces furunculosis and folliculitis. Both organisms can be associated with impetigo, ecthyma and secondary bacterial infection of scabies and atopic eczema.

Patients with acute erysipelas usually complain of a flu-like illness and may be acutely ill with a high fever, rigors and constitutional upset. The rash consists of a sharply demarcated fiery erythema. Oedema is often prominent, and petechiae or haemorrhagic blisters may form. The lower leg is the site most commonly involved although erysipelas may also been seen affecting the face, arm and buttock.

It is certain that Group A beta-haemolytic streptococci are the commonest organisms to cause erysipelas. Group B, C and G streptococci have also been associated with the disease; rarely *Staphylococcus aureus* can produce a similar picture.

Penicillin is unquestionably the drug of choice for erysipelas. Ideally it should be given parenterally until the patient has been apyrexial for 48 hours (e.g. 600 mg IM or IV every 6 hours). A further 2 weeks of oral penicillin should then be prescribed. Broad-spectrum antibiotics, such as ampicillin, are not so effective. Erythromycin is the second line drug for penicillin sensitive patients.

Recurrent erysipelas is a more difficult problem usually affecting the face or leg. There may be an obvious 'portal of entry' for the streptococcus such as a leg ulcer, or chronic tinea pedis, which should be closed. If this fails prolonged prophylactic antibiotic treatment, e.g. penicillin V 250 mg twice daily orally, should help. Recurrent erysipelas may produce progressive lymphatic obstruction in the leg which should be treated with postural drainage and a support stocking.

Furunculosis or 'boils' are a deep staphylococcal folliculitis. Infection spreads into the perifollicular dermis, resulting in suppuration and necrosis. A carbuncle is a group of furuncles which discharge through several openings. Early furuncles may be aborted by means of antibiotic therapy. If fluctuant, furuncles should be incised and allowed to drain freely. A swab should be taken for bacterial culture and sensitivities. Flucloxacillin or erythromycin are the drugs of choice until sensitivities are available.

A much less troublesome superficial folliculitis can also result from staphyloccocal infection. An example is sycosis barbae, the 'shaving rash' seen in the male beard area. This condition needs to be distinguished from pseudo-sycosis or pseudo-folliculitis barbae. Pseudo-folliculitis can be seen on any hairy site but is particularly troublesome on the beard area of males. Hairs cut with a razor have sharp ends; in curly-haired individuals these can re-enter the skin setting up a 'foreign-body' inflammatory reaction. In Afro-Carribean men the process can go one stage further and produce keloid scarring. Growing a beard will usually control this problem. Using an electric razor and applying clindamycin lotion twice daily may produce some improvement.

Recurrent staphylococcal sepsis does occur and can be very troublesome. The urine of such patients should be tested for the presence of glucose since diabetes mellitus is commonly associated with pyogenic infections. Leukaemia can also present with infections of this type and it is sensible to perform a full blood count. Staphylococci can be 'carried' in the nose and flexures. Regular applications of neomycin and chlorhexidine cream (Naseptin: ICI) will reduce nasal colonization. Daily applications of pHisoMed (Winthrop) to axillae and groin will reduce bacterial colonization in these areas. The pHisoMed, which contains hexachlorophane should be applied for 1–2 minutes before being washed off.

Impetigo is a superficial infection of the skin produced by *Staphylococcus aureus* or, more rarely, this organism in combination with the haemolytic streptococcus. The face is commonly affected and impetigo is predominantly a problem in children. Fragile blisters or pustules form which evolve into the characteristic golden-yellow crusts. Impetigo usually occurs *de novo* but there may be a precipitating cause e.g. scabies, head-lice or atopic eczema.

Children with impetigo should not share towels and face-flannels. It is helpful to remove the crusts once or twice daily after soaking in warm salty water. Most patients receive a topical antimicrobial preparation; neomycin cream or mupirocin ointment (Bactroban: Beecham) would be reasonable choices. I prefer to use a systemic antibiotic. Erythromycin or cephradine (Velosef: Squibb) should be prescribed in doses appropriate to the age of the patient.

Ecthyma is a similar infection. Blisters and pustules form which develop into inflammatory lesions with adherent crusts.

Once the crusts are removed small ulcers remain which eventually heal with scarring. The problem most often involves the lower legs and in Bradford the majority of cases seen are in children recently returned from Pakistan or India. Appropriate systemic and topical antibiotic therapy should be prescribed.

Certain phage group II staphylococci are capable of producing an epidermal cleaving toxin. If these organisms produce impetigo or furunculosis these conditions may be complicated by the staphylococcal scalded skin syndrome (Lyell's syndrome). The almost total shedding of the superficial epidermis presents considerable nursing problems. This complication almost invariably develops in children under 12 who require hospital admission, fluid replacement and parenteral antibiotic therapy. Ultimate recovery is usual.

Gram-negative folliculitis

A facial folliculitis produced by *Proteus* and other Gram-negative organisms can complicate acne treated with multiple systemic antibiotics. Co-trimoxazole or isotretinoin will be effective. Severe cutaneous infections with *Pseudomonas pyocyanea* can afflict patients with immune deficiency. Examples are ecthyma gangrenosum, which can complicate leukaemia, or 'malignant' otitis externa which is seen in elderly diabetics. These are major infections requiring appropriate intravenous antibiotics. Less seriously a pseudomonas folliculitis has been described in the USA in association with the use of 'whirlpool' baths.

Tuberculosis of the skin

Lupus vulgaris (LV) is the classical presentation of cutaneous tuberculosis. Before the availability of milk free from *Mycobacterium tuberculosum* LV was one of the more common chronic skin diseases. Indurated and scarred erythematous plaques develop particularly on the head and neck. Untreated the disease is extremely persistent and destructive. Squamous carcinoma of the skin is a complication of long-standing tuberculous inflammation. Today LV has become quite uncommon and most cases seen are reactivations of old disease. Within the UK I have seen Asian patients with 'cold' subcutaneous tuberculous abscesses, and tuberculous skin ulcers secondary to tuberculous osteomyelitis.

Skin biopsy is usually required to confirm this diagnosis. Samples can be sent for mycobacterial culture although this is often negative. Treatment with rifampicin and isoniazid is usually sufficient to produce resolution of LV. At least 12 months therapy will be necessary. Induration and erythema slowly resolve although pigmentation and some degree of scarring will persist.

Atypical mycobacteria can also infect the skin. Organisms like *Mycobacterium balnei* and *M. ulcerans* grow in fish-tanks and swimming pools. On entering the skin through minor abrasions they produce non-healing ulcers. The organisms may spread up the lymphatics producing sub-cutaneous nodules. Atypical mycobacteria do not respond well to the usual anti-tuberculous drugs but minocycline or co-trimoxazole are often effective.

Erythrasma

This is a chronic, low-grade, infection with *Corynebacterium minutissimum*. The areas affected are the toe-clefts, axillae, sub-mammary skin and the ano-genital region. Patches of infected skin are brown, well-demarcated and slightly scaly. They fluoresce coral red under Woods's light. Erythrasma responds well to sodium fusidate by mouth or miconazole cream.

Practice points

1 *Penicillin is still the treatment of choice for erysipelas.*
2 *There is often a primary underlying cause for extensive impetigo.*
3 *Rarely, any staphylococcal infection can be complicated by the scalded skin syndrome. Hospital admission is essential.*

Virus infections

Warts

Cutaneous warts are the result of infection with the DNA containing human papillomavirus (HPV) (see Plate 2). Several types of wart exist and are produced by different strains of the virus. For example HPV type 1 is associated with deep painful plantar warts (myrmecia); type 2 gives rise to common warts and mosaic plantar warts. HPV type 6 affects the ano-genital region. The replication and maturation of the virus are dependent on substances produced by epidermal cells during keratinization. The immune system mounts a response to the viral infection and consequently there is a high rate of spontaneous remission. It is now recognized that particular genes within the structure of the virus are associated with malignant transformation. It is virtually certain that several HPV types are linked to the development of cervical carcinoma.

Perhaps 30–50% of warts in childhood regress over a 6 months period. The regular use of a salicylic acid paint (e.g. Salactol: Dermal; Duofilm: Stiefel) substantially increases this figure and such preparations should not be regarded merely as placebos. Cryotherapy with liquid nitrogen is widely practised and would normally be considered the treatment of choice for patients whose warts have persisted longer than 6 months despite treatment with topical preparations. Several rather painful sessions are normally required and it should not be employed to treat small, frightened children.

Plantar warts (verrucae) are common and can be single, multiple or mosaic in type. All varieties are covered by a hyperkeratotic cap and it is only after the surface is carefully pared down with a sharp scalpel that the true morphology can be seen. Virus warts contain capillary loops which are visible as red or brown dots and which appear to be surrounded by a horny collar. It may be difficult to distinguish a solitary virus wart from a hard corn. Corns typically occur under the metatarsal heads. If such a corn is pared down no capillary bleeding points are seen but rather a central keratin 'pearl'. Other conditions which occasionally need to be distinguished from warts are the dominantly inherited palmo-plantar callosities, and sub-ungual exostoses. An exostosis is often misdiagnosed as a sub-ungual wart but can be distinguished by its stony hardness and opacity to X-rays.

Plantar warts can be soaked daily in formalin 3% after post bathing abrasion with pumice. The surrounding normal skin is protected with soft paraffin, and the affected area immersed for 10−15 minutes. Six weeks treatment is often required. Alternatively 10% gluteraldehyde (Glutarol: Dermal) or salicylic acid 20% in yellow soft paraffin under adhesive plaster can be applied each day. Mosaic warts are particularly resistant to any form of treatment. Occasionally stubborn warts can be removed by curettage but excision is not generally recommended because of the painful scars that can result. Plane warts on the face are difficult to manage because of the risks of scarring and irritation in a cosmetically crucial site. They are probably best left alone.

ANO-GENITAL WARTS

Ano-genital warts are commonly transmitted by sexual intercourse, indeed genital HPV infection may be the most common sexually transmitted disease. The peak incidence is from the late teens until the early thirties.

There are several morphological presentations including papules, flat warts and the classical 'cauliflower-like' condyloma accuminata. I am sure that ano-genital warts in both sexes are most appropriately treated in departments of genito-urinary medicine. Patients should be screened for other sexually transmitted infections and sexual partners should be checked. The traditional treatment of ano-genital warts is weekly painting with podophyllin 25% in benzoin tincture. The surrounding normal skin is protected with soft paraffin. The podophyllin, which is highly irritating, should be washed off after 4 hours. Cryotherapy is an alternative treatment but resistant anogenital warts may require cautery.

Pregnant women may experience rapid growth of vulval condyloma accuminata which become painful and offensive. Podophyllin is contra-indicated during pregnancy. Cryotherapy or cautery are possible but the management of such patients should be discussed with an obstetrician. HPV is believed to be essentially 'site specific'. Babies may be infected from their mother's genital tract during delivery and will themselves develop ano-genital warts within a matter of months. The development of ano-genital warts by older children raises the possibility of child sexual abuse.

MOLLUSCUM CONTAGIOSUM

The pearly umbilicated papules of this pox virus infection contain myriads of virus particles. The disease is usually seen in children, where the face and axillae are common sites, and young adults where perigenital lesions are frequent. Quite severe infections can develop in atopics. Inflammation of the papules usually leads to rapid resolution. This fact has been exploited in treatment strategies:
• Pricking with a pointed stick.
• Lightly freezing with liquid nitrogen.
• Squeezing with fine forceps.
Cryotherapy with liquid nitrogen is my preferred treatment but in fact none of these measures are practical in apprehensive small children. If a group of mollusca are close together the application of EMLA cream (Astra) for 1−2 hours prior to cryotherapy should produce sufficient analgesia to permit the procedure. Since there is almost always spontaneous resolution in 12−18 months a painless placebo is preferable in young children.

Herpes simplex

Recurrent perioral herpes simplex or 'cold sores' is a familiar disorder. Primary infection in early childhood normally causes a gingivo-stomatitis although severe primary infections of the facial or perioral skin are also seen. Herpes simplex virus type 1 (HSV1) is usually responsible for these presentations; it can however also be isolated from genital lesions. HSV2 is almost exclusively associated with the anogenital pattern of herpes, which is becoming increasingly common, and also with

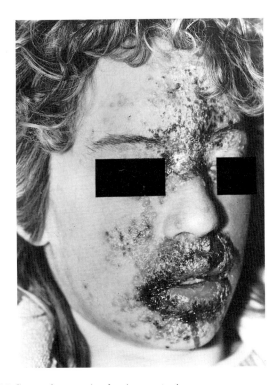

Fig. 5.13 Severe herpes simplex in an atopic

generalized infection in the neonatal period.

Infections at other sites, such as the fingers or buttocks, may be more difficult to recognize because of their unfamiliarity. Typical infection produces painful or itchy vesicular lesions which recur at the same site on several occasions and persist for 10−14 days.

Recurrent perioral cold sores are seldom a major problem and painting with an antiseptic (e.g. povidone−iodine) is satisfactory. Several specifically antiviral topical preparations are available. Two examples are idoxuridine 5% in dimethyl sulphoxide (Herpid: WB Pharmaceuticals) and acyclovir 5% cream (Zovirax: Wellcome). Clearly neither product would be indicated unless the attacks were frequent and severe. Patients should commence treatment as soon as possible after the onset of prodromal symptoms. Trials of acyclovir cream have not been unanimous in attributing benefits to this preparation. By contrast the continuous oral use of acyclovir in a dose of 200 mg four times daily is effective, in about 75% patients, for suppressing recurrent perioral and genital herpes. The cost of continuous oral acyclovir treatment will restrict its use to those with very severe episodes or post-viral erythema multiforme. Episodic herpes simplex returns once therapy is discontinued.

Oral, or even parenteral, acyclovir would be indicated in severe disseminated herpes simplex infections such as those associated with immune deficiency disorders or complicating atopic eczema (Kaposi's eczema herpeticum) (Fig. 5.13). Genital herpes in pregnancy is a special problem since fatal disseminated herpes in the newborn may occur after infection during vaginal delivery. It is agreed that primary genital herpes in the mother is more hazardous that recurrent disease but both may be clinically silent. Babies exposed to primary herpes simplex during delivery should be treated with acyclovir.

Herpes zoster

Herpes zoster or shingles is caused by the reactivation of latent varicella-zoster virus present in sensory dorsal root cells since an earlier attack of chickenpox (Fig. 5.14). The names 'shingles' and 'zoster' derive from the words for 'belt' respectively in Latin and Greek. Shingles may develop in any dermatome; normally the disease is characterized by pain and a vesicular rash but either feature can occur in isolation.

Ultimately shingles will affect one adult in twenty. The disease can affect all age groups but is more common in the elderly and it is this group that is most frequently afflicted by post-herpetic neuralgia. Involvement of the naso-ciliary branch of the trigeminal nerve results in ophthalmic zoster. This complication should be anticipated if vesicles develop on the upper part of the nose; major eye damage may follow and early advice from an ophthalmologist is essential.

In young, and otherwise healthy, subjects analgesia and

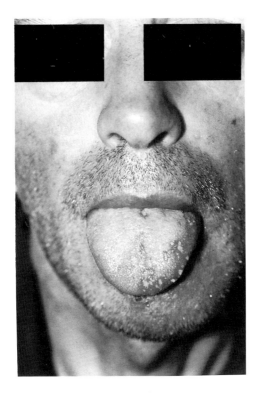

Fig. 5.14 Herpes zoster effecting left side of tongue

antiseptics are sufficient treatment for an attack of herpes zoster. In severely affected individuals it may be impossible to give adequate analgesia without resort to opiates. Patients over 60 years are more prone to develop post-herpetic neuralgia. Acyclovir in a dose of 800 mg five times daily for 7 days reduces acute pain and possibly the incidence of neuralgia.

Established post-herpetic neuralgia is a most intractable and demoralizing problem. Most patients will benefit from the special expertise of a pain clinic. Simple analgesics are seldom, if ever, effective but combinations of tricyclic antidepressants and phenothiazines have been beneficial. An example is amitriptyline and perphenazine (Triptafen DA: Allen & Hanburys). Some drug resistant patients have improved following the use of transcutaneous nerve stimulation.

Orf

This rural zoonosis is the infection of humans with the paravaccinia virus that causes contagious pustular dermatosis of sheep. Inflamed, purplish and blistered areas occur on the fingers, and occasionally other exposed sites. Spontaneous remission is usual. Antiseptics and systemic antibiotics should prevent secondary bacterial infection.

Hand, foot and mouth disease

This condition is caused by the virus Coxsackie A16. It usually affects young children and often is seen in minor epidemics. Fragile greyish blisters or pustules develop on the fingers, toes and occasionally other sites. Mouth ulcers are frequent although systemic upset is rare. Spontaneous recovery with lasting immunity will occur over 10–14 days. The disorder is unrelated to foot and mouth disease of sheep.

Practice points

1 *Eczema herpeticum affects atopic patients producing profuse inflammatory blistering involving the head and upper trunk.*
2 *Ano-genital warts in both sexes are most appropriately treated in departments of genito-urinary medicine.*
3 *Patient's with ophthalmic herpes zoster require urgent referral to an ophthalmologist.*

Fungal and yeast infections

Dermatophyte infections

Few fungi are pathogenic to man; most are saprophytes obtaining their nutrients by the degradation of dead organic material. Essentially we are concerned with superficial infections produced by the dermatophyte, or ringworm producing, fungi. In the UK the genera predominantly involved are *Trichophyton*, *Microsporum* and *Epidermophyton* (Table 5.6).

Dermatophytes invade the keratin of the hair, skin and

Table 5.6   Origin of fungal species

T. rubrum	Human
T. violaceum	Human
T. mentagrophytes	Animal
T. interdigitale	Human
T. verrucosum	Animal
M. canis	Animal
M. gypseum	Soil-inhabiting
E. floccosum	Human

nails. Depending on the species involved a variable inflammatory response is elicited from the host. This may be modest (lesions dry and scaly) or marked (lesions erythematous and vesicular). Dermatophyte infections are normally described as 'tinea' followed by the anatomical site involved e.g. scalp ringworm = tinea capitis, foot ringworm = tinea pedis.

Tinea capitis is almost exclusively seen in children. The zoophilic cat ringworm fungus (*Microsporum canis*) causes a patch of scarring alopecia with scaling and broken hairs. Children can develop a more inflammatory scalp ringworm resulting from infection with the fungus *Trichophyton violaceum*. The species has been noted among Asian communities in London and Bradford.

Cattle ringworm (*T. verrucosum*) infection of the scalp is naturally commoner in rural areas. The resulting infection (kerion) is pustular and inflammatory with marked hair loss. It most commonly affects the scalp in childhood but can cause tinea barbae in adult males. Under the microscope the spores of trichophyton species are actually within hair shafts, an appearance described as endothrix. Conversely the spores of microsporum species are noted to aggregate around hair shafts (ectothrix).

Patients with tinea corporis develop scaly erythematous rings showing central clearing and sometimes peripheral vesiculation (Fig. 5.15). In tinea cruris similar lesions extend out from the inguinal area. This problem is almost entirely restricted to adult men and is usually associated with tinea pedis. Tinea pedis is probably the commonest dermatophyte infection. It is variable in extent from simple interdigital

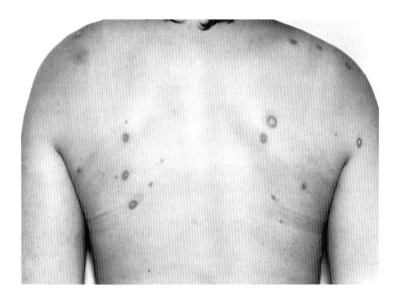

Fig. 5.15 Annular lesions of tinea corporis

infection (Athlete's foot) to extensive erythema and scaling.

Nail plate invasion by dermatophytes (tinea unguium) is commoner in toenails than finger nails (see Plate 3). Onycholysis is often an early feature but eventually the affected nail plates become thickened, distorted and yellowish. A feature that is of value in distinguishing tinea unguium from other causes of nail dystrophy, such as that of psoriasis, is that fungal infection produces asymmetrical nail involvement.

Dermatophyte fungi can often be succesfully cultured from affected hair or skin. The fungi are easily visible if skin scrapings mounted in 10% potassium hydroxide solution are examined microscopically. Scalp hairs infected with *M. canis* show a turquoise fluorescence if examined in Wood's light.

The imidazoles (clotrimazole, miconazole etc) are non-irritating, cosmetically acceptable and have a broad-spectrum of activity. Most fungal infections of glabrous skin will respond to twice daily application for 3–4 weeks. Infections of the scalp, or extensive and resistant infections at any site, should in addition be treated with oral griseofulvin (Fulcin: ICI). For an adult a dose between 500–1000 mg daily, with fatty food, is normally sufficient. For the occasional adult patient who cannot tolerate griseofulvin, itraconazole (Sporanox: Janssen) can be prescribed:

Tinea corporis/cruris	100 mg daily for 15 days
Tinea manum/pedis	100 mg daily for 30 days
Tinea unguium	Not recommended

Scalp infection in children requires 8–12 weeks treatment with griseofulvin elixir in a weight related dose (10 mg/Kg). A topical antifungal will not eradicate scalp ringworm but may lessen the chance that the infection will be disseminated. Children should be kept away from school for the first 2–3 weeks of treatment. Fungal infection of a finger nail plate requires griseofulvin treatment for 6 months while the damaged nail plate 'grows out'. Toe nail involvement may not clear with even 12–18 months of continuous treatment. Realistically only a 50% cure rate can be anticipated. Patients with nail dystrophy should not be prescribed systemic antifungal agents unless a fungus has been seen or cultured.

Trosyl nail solution (Pfizer) can be painted on the affected nails twice daily until no visibly affected plate is left. Avulsion of severely affected nail plates may shorten the duration of treatment. As an alternative to surgical removal 40% urea paste can be applied to the affected nail plates under an occlusive dressing for 10–14 days. The affected parts of the plate soften and can easily be removed with scissors and forceps whilst the normal, uninvaded, portion of the nail plate is unaffected.

Practice points

1 *Nystatin cream is only effective against the yeast* Candida albicans, *and not against the true fungi.*
2 *Dermatophyte infections of the scalp require griseofulvin therapy and will not respond to topical antifungals alone.*

Pityriasis versicolor

Pityriasis versicolor is a common, and frequently symptomless,

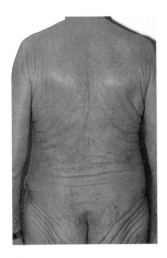

Plate 1 Erythrodermic eczema.

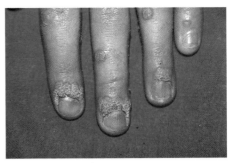

Plate 2 Extensive periungual warts.

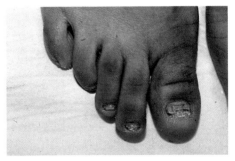

Plate 3 Fungal invasion of nail plates; tinea unguim.

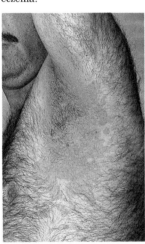

Plate 4 (*Left*) Pityriasis versicolor; a symptomless yeast infection.

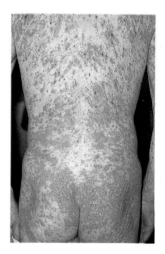

Plate 5 Extensive lichen planus.

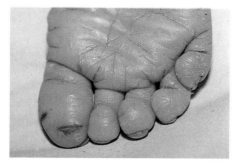

Plate 6 Juvenile plantar dermatosis.

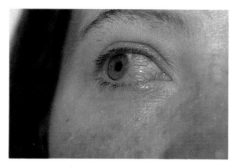

Plate 7 Rosacea of cheek with eye involvement.

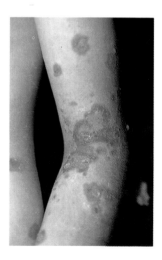

Plate 9 Extensive impetigo secondary to scabies.

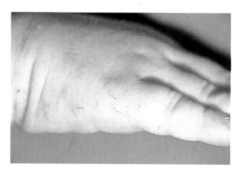

Plate 8 Scabies; prominent burrows.

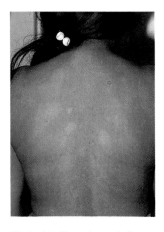

Plate 10 Hypopigmented patches in borderline leprosy.

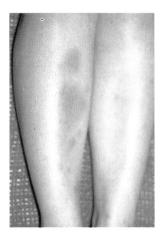

Plate 11 Post-streptococcal erythema nodosum.

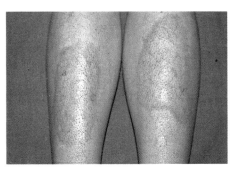

Plate 12 Necrobiosis lipoidica.

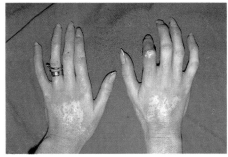

Plate 13 Systemic sclerosis involving hands.

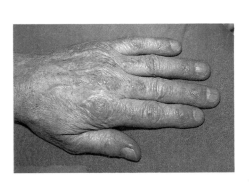

Plate 15 Polymorphic eruption of pregnancy.

Plate 14 (*Left*) Dermatomyositis: knuckle and nail fold changes.

infection of the stratum corneum by the yeast *Pityrosporum orbiculare* (see Plate 4). The rash usually affects the trunk and upper arms. There are approximately annular pink or tancoloured macules which may be confluent. Fine scaling is visible if the lesions are abraded. Infection commonly leads to macular hypopigmentation of the skin. This is very obvious in Asian patients but in whites becomes visible only after sunbathing. This hypopigmentation may persist for months after successful treatment and should not be interpreted as a relapse.

Pityrosporum orbiculare cannot be cultured using ordinary techniques but spores and hyphae are easily visible on microscopic examination of skin scrapings. Any imidazole antifungal will control this infection if applied nightly to all affected areas for 10–14 days, although relapses are frequent. Systemic treatment should be reserved for the few patients with very extensive disease or those who relapse quickly after apparently successful topical therapy. Suitable regimes are:
- Ketoconazole 200 mg daily for 14 days.
- Itraconazole 200 mg daily for 7 days.

Practice points

1 *The organism responsible for pityriasis versicolor is sensitive neither to nystatin nor griseofulvin.*
2 *After successful treatment hypopigmentation may persist for months and should not be interpreted as a relapse.*

Candidiasis

Oral candidiasis is popularly known as 'thrush'; candida can also cause an erythematous pustular intertrigo, vulvo-vaginitis, or balanitis. In these sites a bright red primary lesion with satellite pustules is usual. Between the fingers candida can produce macerated skin with patches of denudation, an appearance described as erosio interdigitale. It is important to identify a predisposing cause if one exists:
- diabetes
- pregnancy
- drug treatment:

steroids
broad-spectrum antibiotic
- immune deficiency disorder

Imidazoles are rapidly effective against candida. For vaginal thrush an econazole pessary inserted on three successive nights together with econazole cream applied twice daily is a highly effective regime. Nystatin is not absorbed after oral administration but 500 000 units given four times daily for 5 days would eradicate the reservoir of organisms in the gut. Candida vulvo-vaginitis and balanitis are frequently transmitted sexually. It is therefore essential to treat sexual partners. Any patients with genital candida infection should have their urine tested for glucose.

Chronic paronychia is an infection of the space between the nail plate and the posterior nail fold with candida and bacteria. It is common in women who frequently immerse their hands in water hence the old name of 'bar-maids disease'. The cuticle is lost, the nail plate is often dystrophic and the posterior nail fold is red, swollen and may discharge pus. Management is difficult since it is necessary to keep the finger dry at all times. Rubber gloves or a finger stall should be worn. An antimicrobial agent which penetrates the nail fold well should be applied 4–6 times daily. An imidazole lotion such as clotrimazole or econazole can be employed but inevitably the treatment takes many weeks. Griseofulvin is frequently prescribed for this disorder but cannot possibly help since the organisms involved are not dermatophyte fungi.

Chronic paronychia can be punctuated by episodes of acute, usually staphylococcal, infection. The periungual area becomes more painful and swollen. A bead of pus may be expressible from the posterior nail fold. This complication should be treated with systemic antibiotics. Incision of the nail fold will only serve to further damage the disturbed architecture of the region.

Practice points

1 Candida albicans *commonly causes secondary infection of napkin eruptions. Treat both problems concurrently.*
2 *Chronic paronychia is unresponsive to griseofulvin.*

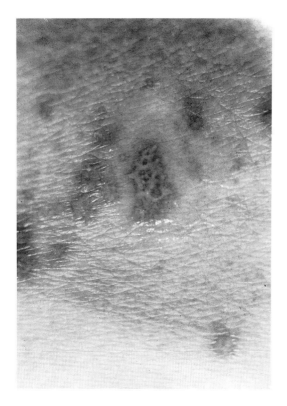

Fig. 5.16 Lichen planus showing Wickham's striae

Lichen planus

Lichen planus is an inflammatory disorder of the skin characterized by a pruritic, purple, polygonal papular rash (Fig.
5.16) (see Plate 5). The wrists and forearms are usually involved but any area can be affected. Involvement of the lips,
buccal mucosa and glans penis is seen frequently. The disease
often shows the Köbner phenomenon. If the disease exhibits
marked involvement of hair follicles it is termed lichen plano-
pilaris. This variety is commonly associated with scalp involvement which can result in scarring alopecia. Eventually
spontaneous resolution of lichen planus occurs and residual
pigmentation is very prominent.

The cause of lichen planus is unknown but the primary event is probably an attack on the epidermis by activated T-lymphocytes. A virtually identical rash may be part of graft v. host disease following bone marrow transplantation. Localized lichen planus responds best to potent topical steroid treatment, with or without polythene occlusion. Antihistamines may help the severe pruritus. If the rash is very extensive treatment with sytemic steroids may be considered necessary. A reasonable initial dose for an adult would be prednisolone 30 mg daily for 2 weeks, decreasing to zero very gradually over 8–12 weeks. Systemic steroids certainly suppress the pruritus and rash; it is much less certain that the natural history of the disease is altered.

The lace-like buccal lesions of lichen planus are usually asymptomatic and are often not noted by the patient. In the uncommon ulcerative or erosive form mouth lesions can be sore and interfere with eating.

Practice points

1 *For diagnosing lichen planus remember the 'Ps': pruritic, purple, polygonal and, ultimately, pigmented.*
2 *Post-inflammatory pigmentation after lichen planus is very obvious indeed in brown or black skinned patients.*

Nail disorders

ONYCHOGRYPHOSIS

Onychogryphosis is thickening and twisting of the nail plate which most commonly affects the toes of the elderly. Trauma, self-neglect and perhaps circulatory impairment are responsible.

BRITTLE AND SPLIT NAILS

Brittleness is a common complaint although often there is no obvious cause. It can be a feature of iron deficiency or be related to exposure to substances such as detergents and solvents. Brittleness can be the end point of many skin disorders that involve the nail plate. In lamellar nail dystrophy the distal portion of the nail splits into thin plates. The disorder is usually seen in adult women and is thought to relate to water and detergent exposure.

ONYCHOLYSIS

Onycholysis represents symptomless separation of the nail plate from the nail bed. Classically this is seen in psoriasis although it may also be a feature of fungus infections, phototoxic drug eruptions and hyperthyroidism. Idiopathic onycholysis is occasionally seen, usually in middle-aged women with long nails. Leverage from the long nails is certainly a contributory, and perhaps the only, cause. In all patients with onycholysis trimming back the nails is essential.

PITTING

Pitting is the commonest nail plate abnormality. Psoriasis is a common cause but pits may also occur if there is an eczematous rash on the fingers. When fine nail pitting occurs in association with alopecia areata it is a poor prognostic sign.

RIDGING

Beau's lines are transverse depressions which develop across the nail plates following severe skin or systemic illnesses. Any disorder that interferes with activity of the nail matrix can produce this sign which becomes visible once the nail growth resumes. Multiple transverse depressions can follow repeated trauma to the cuticle and nail fold as is seen in the 'habit tic' type of nail dystrophy.

Disorders of the perinychial tissues

Chronic paronychia has been dealt with in the section on fungal and yeast diseases. Virus warts are frequently found in the periungual area. They seem more resistant than usual to the curative properties of wart paints and cryotherapy is particularly painful in this region. Mucoid or myxoid cysts are generally found on the posterior nail folds of the fingers. They are dome shaped and are often associated with a longitudinal depression of the nail plate. The disorder is a degenerative change originating from the underlying phalangeal joint. Cryotherapy, excision and intralesional triamcinolone injection can all be effective but recurrence is frequent whatever form of treatment is adopted.

Practice points

1 *Fungal nail disease is the easiest to cure. Whatever the appearance of the dystrophic nail it is never wrong to examine nail fragments microscopically for fungal hyphae.*
2 *Pitting is the commonest nail plate abnormality and is not specific to psoriasis.*

Oral disease

Aphthous ulceration

Mild ulceration can be helped by a soluble salicylate gel (e.g. Bonjela: Reckitt & Colman). More severe cases can be treated with hydrocortisone 2.5 mg (Corlan: Glaxo) pellets, 4 times daily dissolved in the mouth. More potent topical steroids are also available for oral use such as triamcinolone 0.1% (Adcortyl in Orabase: Squibb) and betamethasone mouth wash. Ten ml of the mouthwash should be held in the mouth for 10 minutes, 3 times daily.

An antibiotic mouth wash can be prepared by dissolving the contents of one 250 mg tetracycline capsule in 10 ml water. This should be used 3 times daily for 3 days. Recently a 1% carbenoxolone preparation has been introduced for this problem (Bioplex: Thames). 2 g of the granules are dissolved in 30 ml water and the result used as a mouth wash 3–4 times daily. Carbenoxolone can promote sodium and water retention, it is important therefore not to swallow the mouth wash. If severe and prolonged, aphthous ulceration can be a very demoralising problem. It may form part of Behçet's syndrome and patients should be questioned about arthralgia, eye symptoms and ano-genital ulceration.

Malignancy

Squamous carcinoma of the lips, tongue and buccal mucosa are not uncommon; suspicious areas must be biopsied early. Squamous carcinoma of the lips is usually the consequence of actinic exposure but can also complicate discoid lupus erythematosus in this region.

Bullous disorders

Oral ulceration is a frequent finding in pemphigus and benign mucous membrane pemphigoid. Systemic steroids are usually required but the problem can be very intractable indeed. Oral ulceration accompanies some cases of erythema multiforme and lichen planus. Topical steroids may be helpful.

Infections

Primary herpetic gingivo-stomatitis can produce marked intra-oral blistering and ulceration. This is usually seen in children who also exhibit profuse salivation and submandibular lymphadenopathy. Ulcerative gingivitis is caused by Vincent's organisms. It requires treatment with antiseptic mouth washes and metronidazole (Flagyl: May & Baker) 200 mg, three times daily for 5 days.

Candida albicans is associated with a number of oral and perioral diseases. Angular stomatitis is a familiar problem. It is normally associated with candida infection although occasionally *Staph. aureus* can produce an identical appearance. Edentulous patients are particularly prone to angular stomatitis. Nystatin cream, or any imidazole, will at least partially control the problem but dental advice is essential. Oral thrush in adults is usually secondary to broad spectrum antibiotic therapy or immuno-suppression. Median rhomboid atrophy of the tongue is now recognized as a chronic form of candidiasis

·and should be treated with long-term nystatin. Nystan pastilles (Squibb) are a pleasant way of administering this drug. Miconazole oral gel is also effective.

Sarcoidosis, tuberculosis, syphilis, fixed drug eruptions and agranulocytosis may all be associated with oral ulceration, although these are rarely encountered in dermatology clinics. A full blood count, serological tests for syphilis, and biopsy for histology and culture should be performed in any patient whose oral ulceration does not have an simple explanation.

Practice points

1 *If patients have severe and recurrent aphthous ulcers, enquire after the other features of Behçet's syndrome.*
2 *Refer for biopsy any patient whose oral ulcer is unexplained.*
3 *If an edentulous patient has chronic candida infection at the angles of the mouth seek the advice of a dentist.*

Paediatric dermatoses

Paediatric dermatology is rapidly developing as a speciality in its own right. Many of the disorders that affect children have been covered in other sections.

- bacterial infections, e.g. impetigo (see p. 76)
- viral infections, e.g. warts, molluscum contagiosum (see p. 81)
- infestations, e.g. scabies, head lice (see p. 125)
- atopic eczema (see p. 56)
- ichthyosis (see p. 73)
- guttate psoriasis (see p. 113)

In this section I shall discuss the following disorders not described elsewhere:

- vascular birthmarks
  strawberry naevus
  portwine stain
  salmon patch
- toxic erythema of the newborn
- epidermolysis bullosa

- napkin eruptions
- juvenile plantar dermatosis
- granuloma annulare

Vascular naevi

The capillary haemangioma, or strawberry naevus, is a red lobulated tumour that develops rapidly in the first few weeks of life. Girls are affected more frequently than boys. The head, particularly the central face, and trunk are common sites for this lesion. After a period of active growth lasting a year or so the strawberry naevus ultimately involutes with fibrosis. By the age of 8–10 residual scarring is frequently minimal. Unless the eye or airway are involved in early infancy attempts at intervention are best avoided. On the rare occasions that treatment is required systemic steroids will produce shrinkage. Bleeding from strawberry naevi can be simply controlled with pressure.

The well-known naevus flammeus, or portwine strain, is present at birth and seldom, if ever, shows significant involution. Excision of port wine stains is rarely practical. Treatment with the argon or tuneable dye laser is lengthy and tedious. Benefits, in adults at least, can be impressive although due to the expense of the equipment it will be some time before this type of treatment is widely available in the UK. Results from cosmetic camouflage can be very good indeed and this form of management should be offered to all affected patients. The salmon patch is commonly called the 'stork mark'. It is an area of macular erythema found on the nape of the neck or forehead. Salmon patches on the neck persist; those on other sites fade during infancy.

Toxic erythema of the newborn

This disorder is seen during the first week of life and consists of an erythematous macular rash. In the centre of the macules there are eosinophil containing pustules. The disorder is of no significance and settles quickly without treatment.

Epidermolysis bullosa (EB)

EB represents a complex group of genetically determined primary bullous disorders of the skin. In general dominantly inherited variants are less severe than those inherited recessively; splitting occurs through the basal layer of the epidermis or at the dermo-epidermal junction. Blistering follows trauma to the skin and, if not actually present at birth, develops during the first year of life. EB can be classified clinically on the basis of the family history, the severity of the disease and the involvement of teeth or nails. The diagnosis can be made more precise by the examination of a skin biopsy under the electron microscope to determine the exact level of splitting.

At present no curative treatment exists for any type of EB. Patients may be helped by the avoidance of trauma and the prevention of secondary infection. There is a very active and helpful patients' organisation within the UK. Some centres can perform prenatal skin biopsy if mothers have previously given birth to a severely disabled child.

Napkin eruptions

There is now general agreement that the true 'napkin dermatitis' is an irritant and frictional eczema produced by prolonged contact with urine soaked nappies (Fig. 5.17). The problem is at least made worse by the use of polythene pants. A glazed erythema with erosions is characteristic (Jaquet's erythema). The flexures, protected from exposure, are usually spared. This type of problem is becoming less common following the widespread adoption of disposable nappies.

Some infants have a rash affecting the whole napkin area with no flexural sparing. Seborrhoeic eczema of infancy presents as a diffuse, erythematous shiny or greasy rash extending out from the groin. Involvement of the other flexures together with 'cradle cap' are also common. 'Psoriasiform' napkin eruption usually presents in the first 4 months of life and is more resistant to treatment. Well demarcated erythematous plaques are covered in a silvery scale that resembles psoriasis. The limbs, face and scalp may also be involved. The exact status of

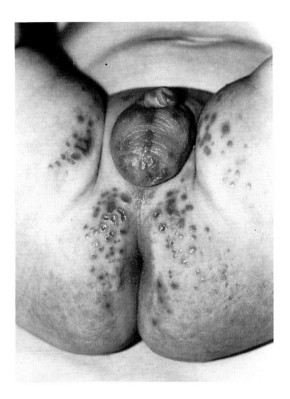

Fig. 5.17 An erosive 'napkin dermatitis'

these two disorders is far from clear. A substantial portion of infants with seborrhoeic eczema of infancy develop atopic eczema in later life. A smaller proportion with psoriasiform napkin eruption ultimately develop classical psoriasis. Many children in both groups have no skin problems after infancy. Napkin eruptions in Asian or Afro-Caribbean children may be complicated by marked, but temporary, depigmentation.

The successful treatment of any napkin eruption requires the full co-operation of the parents. Wet nappies should be changed as frequently as reasonably possible. The baby's skin should be scrupulously cleaned with oil or plain warm water. Washed nappies should be thoroughly rinsed to ensure that they do not contain residues of soap or detergent. It goes without saying that 'grey' nappies are not being adequately laundered.

In early mild napkin dermatitis the use of a simple protective preparation such as dimethicone cream, or zinc and castor oil cream, is usually sufficient. More severe rashes are commonly infected secondarily with *Candida albicans* or *Staphylococcus aureus*. Here a hydrocortisone or antimicrobial preparation is valuable. An example would be a cream containing chlorhexidine, nystatin and hydrocortisone (Nystaform-HC Cream: Bayer) applied 3 times daily. Potent topical steroids are contra-indicated in this situation. There is a risk of skin atrophy, worsening infection and the development of the so-called infantile gluteal granuloma. These are nodular lesions, somewhat reminiscent of haemangiomas. Some consider them to be the result of candida super-infection.

The seborrhoeic and psoriasiform eruptions can initially be treated in the same way although the psoriasiform pattern is slow to respond to any treatment. Two percent salicylic acid in Unguentum Merck may help break up the greasy adherent scales on the scalp and a hydrocortisone or urea cream (Calmurid-HC: Pharmacia) may be helpful. Widespread secondary infection with staphylococci should be treated with a systemic antibiotic.

Practice points

1 *Give advice and emollients before topical steroids.*
2 *If topical steroids are necessary use hydrocortisone preparations.*
3 *Do not use potent fluorinated steroids at all.*

Juvenile plantar dermatosis

Juvenile plantar dermatosis (JPD) occurs between the ages of 5 and 15. Scaling and painful fissuring is seen on the tips of the toes, or more generally over the forefoot (see Plate 6). Overall the skin has a glazed and shiny appearance. JPD seems to be a genuinely new disease with the first cases reported in the mid-1970s. It is often misdiagnosed as a fungus infection but the actual cause is uncertain. It is not a straightforward contact dermatitis but nevertheless may in some way be produced by the materials used to make modern shoes and socks. Topical steroids are unhelpful but simple emollients may produce partial improvement. Some children benefit from the substitution of leather shoes for 'trainers', and woollen socks for fluorescent nylon.

Granuloma annulare

Granuloma annulare (GA) is an inflammatory disorder of dermal collagen (Fig. 5.18). The aetiology is unknown. Lesions consist of firm, flesh-coloured papules which often coalesce to form the characteristic ring-like appearance. GA usually affects children and young adults. The hands and feet are sites of predilection but rarely it may occur elsewhere. Solitary lesions are occasionally mistaken for ringworm. GA is normally symptomless and self-limiting and does not require treatment in childhood. Potent topical steroids may sometimes hasten resolution in adults at the risk of producing skin atrophy.

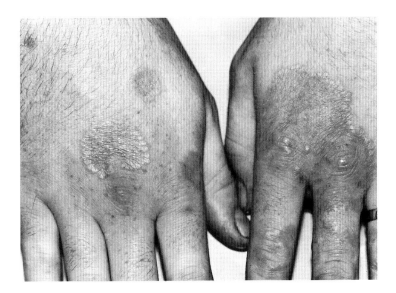

Fig. 5.18 Granuloma annulare

Photosensitivity

Despite the widespread acceptance of the concept among the fashion conscious there is, in reality, no such thing as a 'healthy tan'. The unprotected pale skin of the fair and red-headed members of the population is particularly vulnerable to actinic damage. In normal individuals the acute adverse effects of excessive sun exposure are of course the familiar triad of pain, erythema and oedema known as sunburn.

The wrinkling, yellowness and telangiectasia which form the features of premature skin aging are certainly signs of long-standing sun exposure. There is overwhelming evidence that solar keratoses and most non-melanoma skin cancers are related to a lifetime total dose of ultraviolet irradiation.

Photosensitivity normally affects exposed sites such as the face, forearms, backs of the hands, and the lower legs (particularly in women and children). The areas underneath the chin and behind the ears are characteristically spared. The morphology of the rash depends on the cause of the photosensitivity but erythema, scaling, urticarial wheals and blisters are all possible. In northern England the 'season' for photosensitivity is from April to September.

Phototoxicity, in theory, occurs in all individuals exposed to sufficient doses of both the phototoxic agent and the appropriate radiation. It can occur on first exposure. It is not an immune response and produces a fairly uniform erythema on exposed areas.

The majority of the drug induced phototoxic responses result in sensitivity to UVA.

- amiodarone
- Phenothiazines
- nalidixic acid
- Psoralens
- Thiazides, e.g. hydrochlorothiazide
- Sulphonamides, including sulphonylureas
- tetracyclines, e.g. demethylchlortetracycline
- Quinine
- quinidine

   Contact photoallergy involves the immune system, it cannot

occur on first exposure to the agent concerned. Clinically the reaction resembles a dermatitis and is patchy. Allergic contact dermatitis and photoallergic contact dermatitis can occur alone or in combination and can produce a variety of clinical changes.

Photoallergy can result from contact with:
- halogenated salicylanilides, and other antimicrobials
- hexachlorophane
- perfumes, especially musk ambrette
- sunscreens
- plants, e.g. compositae or umbelliferae
- tar products
- dyes
- phenothiazines and sulphonamides

Excessive alcohol consumption, or occasionally oestrogens, can cause photosensitivity by inducing aquired hepatic cutaneous porphyria (porphyria cutanea tarda). Skin on exposed areas such as the face and backs of the hands becomes fragile. Blisters form which characteristically heal with milia formation. Hypertrichosis may develop. There are typical skin biopsy features and the excretion of urinary uroporphyrins is raised. Treatment includes strict alcohol avoidance and small doses of antimalarials, such as Chloroquine 200 mg twice *weekly*. Resistant patients may respond to regular venesection which helps by reducing body iron stores.

Erythropoietic protoporphyria (EPP) is not drug induced but may also produce an extreme photosensitivity in childhood. This metabolic abnormality is inherited as an autosomal dominant. Affected children characteristically have small pitted scars on the nose; high levels of erythrocyte protoporphyrin are present in the blood.

The commonest idiopathic photodermatosis is polymorphic light eruption (PLE). Affected patients, who are usually adult females, develop erythema, papules and itching on exposed sites. PLE is not usually a very severe problem but can persist for years. A more extreme form of photosensitivity, actinic reticuloid, affects elderly men.

Few of the diseases mentioned are curable. For the majority of patients sun-avoidance and high protection factor sunscreens are essential. Unfortunately all sunscreens are better able to protect normal individuals from excessive exposure than they are able to protect the genuinely sun sensitive from even ordinary exposure.

Some patients with EPP have their sun-tolerance improved with betacarotene in doses of up to 200 mg daily. In hospital departments it may be possible to tan photosensitive patients artificially during the winter months so that they are better protected during the Spring and Summer.

SUNBED EXPOSURE

The regular use of 'suntanning beds' by the general public to maintain a suntan is a relatively new phenomenon in the UK and USA. Several patients who have used such sunbeds have been reported to have developed multiple lentigenes somewhat similar to the so-called 'PUVA freckles'. There may also be long-term skin damage. The lack of formal surveillance of such individuals is a matter of concern to many dermatologists and the use of such beds cannot be recommended.

Practice points

1 *If an inflammatory rash is located on exposed sites suspect photosensitivity.*
2 *If photosensitivity is suspected first review the patient's drug therapy.*
3 *Patients with unexplained photosensitivity should be referred to a dermatologist.*

Pigmentary disorders

Disturbance of the skin pigmentation can follow any 'inflammatory' skin disease. Hyperpigmentation is the classical sequel to lichen planus. DLE may cause marked hypo-pigmentation particularly in Afro-Caribbean subjects. Morphoea can present with hypo- or hyperpigmentation. More widespread hyperpigmentation, particularly flexural hyper-pigmentation, is normally associated with an endocrino-logical abnormality (e.g. Addison's disease or thyrotoxicosis) or drug treatment (e.g. chlorpromazine, phenytoin or the antimalarials).

Small areas of idiopathic facial hyperpigmentation are called melasma. This can occur in all ethnic groups but is particularly common in Asian women. Skin bleaches containing hydro-quinone or related substances can be easily purchased from community pharmacists in areas with a large Afro-Caribbean or Asian population. These cannot be recommended because of the risk of inducing hypopigmentation which is even more dis-figuring. Pigmented areas on the face may darken with sun exposure and therefore the regular use of a sunscreen on such sites is reasonable. Remedial cosmetic camouflage is entirely safe and should be offered to all those affected.

Children commonly develop oval or circular hypopigmented patches on the face. This is pityriasis alba which is probably a chronic, low grade, eczema. The disorder affects all ethnic groups but the colour change is obvious only in those of Asian and Afro-Caribbean origin. Ultimately pityriasis alba is self-limiting but it may persist for several years. Salicylic acid 2% ointment or hydrocortisone 1% ointment can be tried.

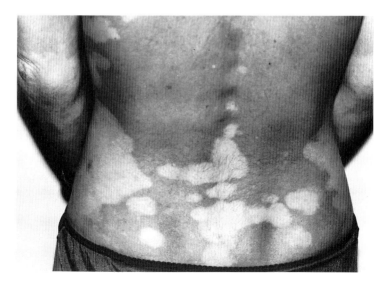

Fig. 5.19 Milk-white patches of vitiligo

Vitiligo affects perhaps 1% of the population (Fig. 5.19). In this condition there is destruction, probably autoimmune destruction, of melanocytes in the basal layer of the epidermis. As a result symmetrical depigmented patches develop with the face, limbs, and trunk all being commonly affected. Occasionally vitiligo remits spontaneously but most patients exhibit a slowly progressive course. Apart from the appearance and the inevitable sensitivity to sunlight the affected areas of skin are entirely normal.

On the untanned skin of white skinned people patches of vitiligo are scarcely perceptible although visability is aided by examination in Wood's light. In such patients the skin is either normal or totally white. In Afro-Caribbean or Asian patients partially involved areas may also be seen giving an appearance described as 'trichrome' vitiligo. The disorder is of very profound significance in dark skinned people. It represents a very obvious cosmetic disability and patients often receive the diagnosis with considerable alarm.

Some Muslim patients believe the disease is acquired by eating milk, fish and other white foods. Many will have already been advised by relatives to abstain from white foodstuffs (e.g. milk, yoghurt, and egg white) and may be using traditional remedies such as holy water or sand from Mecca. Old Hindu traditions may regard vitiligo as a punishment incurred for sins committed in a previous life. It is difficult to exaggerate the hurt and humiliation that vitiligo can inflict and some affected individuals find it almost impossible to maintain any social contacts because of this problem.

Family members show an increased incidence of blood auto-antibodies and related disorders such as alopecia areata, pernicious anaemia and thyrotoxicosis. A very similar occupational leucoderma is encountered in the rubber, plastic and other industries caused by chemicals, such as para-tertiary butyl phenol, which are directly toxic to melanocytes.

Vitiliginous areas may slowly repigment if treated regularly for months with potent fluorinated topical steroid preparations. This will be at the cost of inducing some skin atrophy and this regime should be used with very great caution. PUVA therapy may produce slow peri-follicular repigmentation of vitiliginous areas but the treatment is often unsuccessful while the inevitable darkening of normal skin makes the white patches even more conspicuous. Cosmetic camouflage is the only approach guaranteed to be both safe and helpful. Depigmented patches of skin are sensitive to sun damage and should be protected with a sunscreen.

Practice points

1 *Vitiligo is the cause of great unhappiness. Be sympathetic but not over optimistic about the results of treatment.*
2 *Vitiligo causes depigmentation; pityriasis versicolor, hypopigmentation.*
3 *All patients with pigmentary problems on visible sites should be offered cosmetic camouflage advice.*

Pityriasis rosea

Pityriasis rosea is predominantly a disease of children and young adults (Fig. 5.20). It has long been ascribed to a viral infection but definite proof is lacking. Many patients will have noted an initial larger lesion (the 'herald patch') some days before the typical rash on the trunk develops. White patients develop a profuse, salmon-pink, eruption which affects the neck, trunk and upper arms. Large lesions are oval in shape and some will show a collarette of scales. In Afro-Caribbean patients the rash is more papular, more obviously scaly and darker in colour.

Patients with pityriasis rosea have minimal, if any, constitutional upset and the rash is usually asymptomatic. A few, usually children, develop a more severe problem with facial involvement, fever and lymphadenopathy. In all cases the rash subsides completely within 6−8 weeks and second attacks are extremely uncommon.

Patients require only reassurance and explanation. The few individuals with significant pruritus may be treated with 1% hydrocortisone cream and an antihistamine.

The rash of secondary syphilis can mimic pityriasis rosea quite closely although patients with syphilis will possess

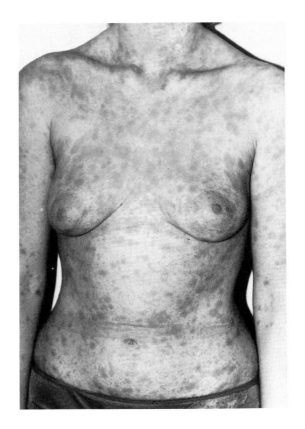

Fig. 5.20 Pityriasis rosea

additional clinical features such as lymphadenopathy, mouth ulcers anc condyloma lata. If there is any doubt serological tests for syphilis should be performed.

Practice points

1 *If a fit young person suddenly develops a macular rash on the trunk with no associated constitutional upset think of pityriasis rosea.*
2 *Pityriasis rosea is not usually itchy but the presence of itching does not eliminate the diagnosis.*

Pruritus

Generalized pruritus

Pruritus is a very common, very demoralizing and very widely misspelt problem. There are many dermatological and medical causes of the symptom but despite extensive investigation a hard core of patients will remain whose itching is totally unexplained.

When confronted with a pruritic patient the first step is to establish whether there is a simple cutaneous cause for the itching. In a individual with no previous history scabies must be the first diagnosis to be considered. Atopic eczema, insect bites, urticaria, lichen planus and dermatitis herpetiformis are all notoriously itchy skin complaints. Xeroderma in the elderly, or contact with fibreglass can both be associated with marked pruritus.

Chronic renal failure is frequently associated with generalized itching although few patients actually present in this way. Infectious hepatitis or any form of obstructive jaundice commonly causes pruritus possibly because of retained bile

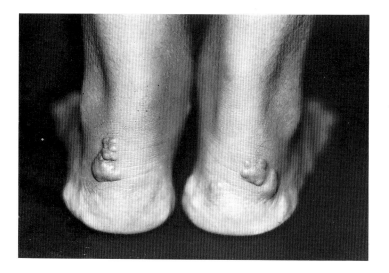

Fig. 5.21 Primary biliary cirrhosis; pruritus and xanthomas

salts (Fig. 5.21). Weight loss, night sweats or lymphadenopathy will suggest the diagnosis of a lymphoma. Pruritus notoriously predates the other symptoms of this disease by months. Poly cythaemia rubra vera can promote major skin irritation particularly after hot bathing.

Generalized pruritus has also been attributed to iron deficiency anaemia, diabetes, hypothyroidism and hyperthyroidism. Although the evidence is less certain these disorders are easy to exclude by simple investigations (Table 5.7). Drug therapy with opiates, phenothiazines or antimalarials may cause extensive itching. Occasionally solid tumours are recognised as being rare causes of pruritus.

The pruritus of lymphoma settles as the patients respond to chemotherapy. Renal transplantation will of course alleviate uraemic pruritus but intractable itching often persists in patients receiving chronic haemodialysis. Parathyroidectomy and ultraviolet irradiation have both been reported as helpful in this situation. The pruritus of partial biliary obstruction may be relieved by the anion exchange resin cholestyramine (Questran: Bristol Myers). Aspirin is said to have a specific effect in relieving the itch of polycythaemia.

Table 5.7   Investigation of generalized pruritus

Examination of skin
General medical examination
Chest X-ray
Urine analysis
FBC and ESR
IgE
Renal function tests
Liver function tests
Thyroid function tests
Blood glucose
Serum protein
electrophoresis

Symptomatic treatment with a sedative antihistamine will usually produce a modest improvement in pruritus. Elderly individuals with xeroderma may improve with emollients and topical steroids. Others may have masked depression that will benefit from the use of tricyclics. Rarely a speculative course of systemic steroids may be justified if the symptom is unendurable, but even then success is not assured.

Practice points

1 *In generalized pruritus first exclude scabies.*
2 *Do not forget the medical causes of pruritus.*

Pruritus ani

Perianal itching is a common symptom and may be the end result of a number of skin complaints including seborrhoeic eczema, flexural psoriasis, tinea, threadworms, lichen sclerosus, warts and contact dermatitis to medicaments. Idiopathic pruritus ani is predominantly a disease of men. Affected patients are often tense, introspective and slightly hostile to a profession that has so obviously failed to control an apparently simple problem. On examination the perianal skin is either normal or simply exhibits the signs of long-standing scratching such as excoriation marks or lichenification.

Treatment should be directed towards establishing optimal anal hygiene; a patient guide is included in Appendix 1. Patch testing may be helpful if an aggravating contact dermatitis to local anaesthetics or topical antihistamines is suspected. It need hardly be added that such remedies should be avoided because of the risks of sensitization; 1% hydrocortisone cream used morning, evening and after each bowel action is often helpful. More potent topical steroids should be avoided in this flexural site. Antihistamines are worth a trial although sedative types such as hydroxyzine (Atarax: Pfizer) are necessary. If all else fails, and it often does, a course of superficial X-ray treatment may help.

Pruritus vulvae

This condition is in many ways the female homologue of the previous complaint. *Candida albicans* and *Trichomonas* may cause vulvo-vaginal soreness and irritation. Vulval lichen planus and lichen simplex (neurodermatitis) of the perivulval skin are relatively easy to recognize, as should be vulval warts and pubic lice. Patients may also develop sensitivity to lubricants or barrier contraceptives. If a specific diagnosis is reached appropriate treatment should be initiated. All patients should be advised to avoid occlusive garments, bubblebaths, irritant soaps and deodorants.

Lichen sclerosus et atrophicus (LSA) results in atrophic porcelain white plaques developing on the ano-genital area, often in a figure of eight arrangement around the vulval and anal orifices. Blistering, often haemorrhagic blistering, is common. Extra-genital lesions are less common but are also white and have a 'cigarette paper' surface. LSA in childhood may resolve spontaneously but the prognosis is much poorer in post-menopausal women. Topical steroids or oestrogens may be of some benefit. Attempts to excise affected areas surgically makes the situation worse.

Vulval pruritus may overlap with vulvodynia or 'burning vulva syndrome' (BVS) although affected women are often very clear that it is soreness or burning they experience, not itching. It is far from clear if BVS is a psychogenic condition, or whether it may have some organic basis. Vestibulitis and human papilloma virus infection have both been linked with this problem. Physical findings are minimal and the response to empirical treatment variable but generally disappointing.

Psoriasis

Psoriasis is a common skin disorder affecting 1–2% of the adult population in the UK. The disease affects both sexes and all ethnic groups, with a peak incidence between the ages of 20–35. Hereditary factors are largely responsibly for the development of the disease, but external factors such as streptococcal infections, stress and drugs (like lithium, beta–blockers and antimalarials) can also be important. There are several clinical patterns:

1 *Chronic plaque* Well defined erythematous plaques are covered in silvery scale. Usually symmetrical with elbows,

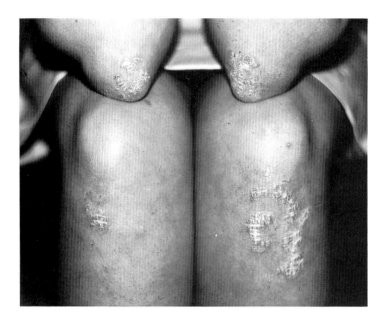

Fig. 5.22 Plaques of psoriasis on the elbows and knees

knees, lower back and scalp being sites of predilection (Fig. 5.22).

2 *Acute guttate* Large numbers of erythematous macules develop over trunk and limbs. This pattern is often post-streptococcal and usually develops in children and young adults.

3 *Flexural* Flexural involvement is common in plaque psoriasis although some patients have exclusively flexural disease. Flexural plaques are moist rather than scaly but retain their well defined character.

In chronic plaque psoriasis dithranol (*USA Anthralin*) is still an effective treatment for most patients. The celebrated British dermatologist J.T. Ingram devised a regime which has been successfully used for many years:

- clean off old paste with oil
- soak in tar bath for 20 minutes
- descale lesions with a towel
- give sub-erythema dose of ultraviolet radiation (UVB)
- apply dithranol in Lassar's paste accurately to each plaque

Initially use a low concentration preparation, e.g. 0.25%. Increase concentration through stage of 0.5%, 1% and 2% depending on patient response.

- dust with zinc oxide or starch powder
- 'suit up' in Tubegauz or Stockinette

Where possible the patient was treated daily; the psoriasis normally regressed in 14−21 days. Treated areas pigmented but on cessation of treatment the pigmentation cleared after 7−10 days.

Over the last 10 years a number of modifications have been made to this regime. The value of the tar bath and UVB have been exaggerated and many centres do not now include them in a standard dithranol regime. Intensive tar and UVB therapy is however a useful method of treatment in itself for some dithranol sensitive patients. Crude coal tar (e.g. 10−20% in yellow soft paraffin) is a reasonably effective substitute for dithranol but is probably too messy for all except hospital in-patients. Ointments containing coal tar solution in soft paraffin are cosmetically more acceptable but less effective than dithranol.

It is now possible to obtain proprietary dithranol prepar-ations in a variety of bases including creams (e.g. Dithrocream: Dermal; Psoradrate: Norwich Eaton) and wax sticks (Antraderm: Brocades). These are more cosmetically acceptable and are readily available from community pharmacies.

The most significant recent improvement in the use of dithranol is the introduction of 'short contact treatment'. This involves increasing the concentration of dithranol applied, but drastically diminishing the exposure time. A suitable regime is given in the appendix. The main benefit is that the patients concerned do not need to have the ointment or paste in contact with their skin for more than 1 to 2 hours each day. Short contact dithranol treatment has been used successfully in hos-pital out-patient clinics but its real advantage is for domestic use.

Scalp psoriasis can be very troublesome and embarrassing. For very mild cases the regular use of a shampoo alone may just be sufficient. Polytar liquid (Stiefel) and Cetavlon-PC (ICI) are popular. More usually an additional topical preparation is necessary. Because of its thickness the scalp is tolerant of topical steroids and daily applications of Synalar Gel (ICI) or Diprosalic Lotion (Kirby-Warwick) can be helpful.

If the scale is thick it is unlikely that these preparations will penetrate. Under these circumstances a greasy preparation containing salicylic acid will be necessary to soften and break up the scale. The hair should be shampooed at night and loose scales combed out. Salicylic acid 2% in Ung. Merck, SCC scalp ointment or a coal-tar and salicylic acid pomade should then be employed. It is essential than the hair should be parted and the preparation applied to the scalp itself. If this treatment is used in the evening the medicament can be left on all night with the patient wearing a shower hat. In the morning the hair is shampooed once more and the scalp is briskly combed to remove as much scale as possible. Ideally this treatment should be repeated nightly until the scalp is clear.

Psoriatic nail dystrophy is common, but effective treatment is rarely possible. Nails should be trimmed as short as possible as leverage can worsen onycholysis.

Flexural or facial psoriasis should not be treated with dithranol which is too irritating for use on these sites. Topical steroid preparations are helpful but great care must be exercised in the use of these preparations because of the risk of telangiectasia, flexural atrophy and striae formation. The weakest effective steroid should be used (e.g. Haelan ointment: Dista; Eumovate ointment: Glaxo) and treatment periods made as short as possible. Sadly there still seem to be patients who are being prescribed large quantities of potent topical steroids as the sole treatment of psoriasis. The great risk is the development of an unstable erythematous form of the disease which thereafter proves difficult to manage by any safer means.

Guttate psoriasis is commoner in children, particularly following streptococcal infections. It usually resolves within a few months irrespective of therapy. In the early inflammatory stages 1% hydrocortisone cream is safe and soothing. As the guttate lesions become scaly a tar and salicylic acid preparation or Alphosyl-HC cream should be substituted. Recurrent attacks may justify regular prophylactic penicillin, or even tonsillectomy. Affected children frequently develop more classical psoriasis in later life.

The small number of patients with severe, resistant and disabling psoriasis pose a most challenging therapeutic problem. If topical treatment fails completely the use of PUVA, retinoids or cytotoxic drugs can provide acceptable control but there are major adverse effects to be considered. PUVA treatment is clean, easy and pleasant. It produces skin tanning which many patients find attractive. However psoriasis on concealed sites, such as the scalp or crural area, will not respond. Minor side-effects like nausea and pruritus are relatively frequent. It is probable that the overall incidence of non-melanoma skin cancer will be slightly increased in long-term PUVA treated patients. Although the precise mechanism is unknown the retinoid etretinate can unquestionably produce a remission in psoriasis, particularly the erythematous and pustular types. Etretinate has been used alone and in combination with PUVA (RePUVA).

The folic acid antagonist methotrexate (Lederle) is probably the most effective anti-psoriatic agent. Like all anti-metabolites and cytotoxic drugs methotrexate has some major adverse effects and in practice the major limitation on the use of the drug is its tendency to produce hepatic fibrosis, which may lead to cirrhosis. In the treatment of psoriasis single weekly doses between 5–20 mg are used, usually by the oral or intramuscular routes.

Pustular psoriasis

The term is used to describe two distinct conditions. Acute generalized pustular psoriasis is very uncommon; profound constitutional upset is associated with fiery erythema of the skin and sheets of superficial pustulation. A localized pustular skin disease of the palms and soles was previous called pustular psoriasis. Its exact pathogenesis is unknown and the more descriptive term persistent palmo-plantar pustulosis is now preferred (Fig. 5.23). The disease is commoner in women and is characterized by a rash that consists of pustules, bronze-

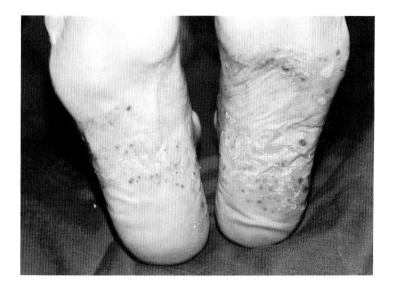

Fig. 5.23 Persistent palmo-plantar pustulosis

coloured macules, and scale. A high percentage of patients have been discovered to be cigarette smokers or to have thyroid dysfunction. Prolonged courses of tetracycline by mouth together with a potent topical steroid may help and is the most practical regimen in young women. Etretinate is more effective but potentially more toxic.

Practice points

1 *No treatment regime for psoriasis represents a cure.*
2 *It is best to provide written instructions for patients prescribed complicated topical treatment regimens.*
3 *Treatment with retinoids or methotrexate should be left to those with special training in their use.*

Raynaud's phenomena and perniosis

Raynaud's phenomena result from paroxysmal constriction of the digital arteries. The pathogenesis is not completely understood; platelet abnormalities, the physical properties of the blood and intrinsic disease of the blood vessels themselves may all contribute.

Clinically pallor of the affected digits is seen which is episodic, bilateral and symmetrical. During an attack pallor is followed by cyanosis, and finally erythema which is the result of reactive hyperaemia. The primary or idiopathic form of the disorder is most commonly seen and can affect the fingers and toes or, more rarely, the nose and ears. There should be no evidence of occlusive vascular disease (Table 5.8).

Table 5.8   Diseases associated with Raynaud's phenomena

Systemic sclerosis
Shoulder girdle compression syndrome
Local circulatory anomalies
Paraproteinaemias and cryoglobulinaemias

Two occupational disorders have features resembling Raynaud's disease. These occur in workers who handle vinyl chloride monomer, and those who work with vibrating-tools like chain saws, power grinders and pneumatic hammers (vibration white finger).

Mild degrees of primary Raynaud's disease are very common indeed; women are affected more frequently than men. The disorder may develop as early as the teens or twenties. Investigation of more severely affected individuals should include full blood count (FBC), anti-nucleur factor (ANF), protein electrophoresis, cryoglobulins and thoracic outlet X-ray.

Raynaud's disease may respond to purely conservative measures. In all but the warmest weather patients should wear thin gloves under thick mittens, together with warm socks and 'sensible' shoes. Smoking should be forbidden in all patients with vascular disease. Existing drug therapy should be reviewed to ensure that beta-blockers or ergot alkaloids are not being prescribed. Electrically heated gloves are available for severely disabled patients (Medmek, PO Box 18, Romsey, Hants). Drugs should be tried in patients with severe symptoms unresponsive to conservative measures and particularly those in whom digital ischaemia actually causes skin infarction.

Vasodilators like thymoxamine (Opilon: Warner) or rheological agents like oxpentifylline (Trental: Hoechst) will provide symptomatic relief in some patients. Cervical sympathectomy may be indicated if the disease is severe enough, if systemic sclerosis is excluded, and no severe secondary changes are present. Unfortunately the improvement tends to be temporary.

Most recently interest has been focused on the use of calcium channel antagonists and in particular nifedipine (Adalat Retard: Bayer). This drug leads to smooth muscle relaxation and is widely reported to be beneficial in Raynaud's phenomenon in doses of 20–40 mg daily. Some patients find the side-effects, like headache, flushing and peripheral oedema, intollerable.

OTHER VASCULAR DISORDERS

Chilblains consist of itchy purplish lumps and are usually seen on the dorsal surfaces of the fingers and toes, particularly in children and young women. Actual ulceration may occur in severe cases. Erythrocyanosis is the name given to the painful itching erythematous plaques that develop on areas of skin exposed to prolonged chilling. The thighs are the commonest sites involved and the typical patient is an obese young woman. Patients who develop blue swollen hands or feet in response to cold are said to have acrocyanosis.

Chilblains and acrocyanosis are relatively common in Asian women probably because the sandals which they wear are quite inadequate protection during a British winter. It seems that shoes are regarded as 'masculine' and are unlikely to be worn although patients may at least be advised to use warm socks. On the whole drug therapy is ineffective and inadvisable.

Buerger's disease is usually seen in relatively young male smokers. Episodic superficial thrombophlebitis occurs, also small vessel occlusions leading to arterial ischaemia. 'Corkscrew' vessels are the typical arteriographic finding.

Practice points
1 *Prevention is better than cure; ensure that gloves and foot-wear are appropriate.*
2 *Stop patients smoking cigarettes. Check that they are not receiving drugs that could exacerbate the problem.*

Rosacea, perioral dermatitis and discoid lupus erythematosus

Rosacea is an inflammatory facial dermatosis of uncertain cause, and variable severity. It is commoner in females with a peak incidence around the ages 30−50. The cheeks, chin and forehead may be involved individually or together. Characteristically pustules and papules are superimposed on a background of erythema and telangiectasia.

Eye complications like blepheritis and keratitis are sometimes seen in patients with rosacea (see Plate 7). A mild degree of lymphoedema is not uncommon in long-standing cases and men often show a degree of sebaceous gland hyperplasia of the nose (rhinophyma). In contrast to acne vulgaris comedones are not seen and the back and chest are uninvolved. The relative rarity of the disorder in the Asian and Afro-Caribbean groups within the UK has resulted in some attributing the disorder to sunlight exposure. Others have blamed a mite, *Demodex folliculorum*, that lives in hair follicles.

In general rosacea responds readily to treatment. Systemic tetracyclines (e.g. Oxytetracycline 250−500 mg twice daily for 12 weeks) are the most valuable drugs. Metronidazole (200 mg twice daily) is a second line agent. The occasional patient who does not respond to either drug may be helped by isotretinoin. Whatever treatment is selected 80% patients require a further course of treatment within 1 year. Topical treatment is of secondary importance. Steroids should never be prescribed but some patients find simple emollients and sunscreens helpful.

Patients with rosacea flush readily. Alcohol, spicy food and temperature changes can exacerbate flushing and patients should be warned to avoid these factors. Flushing and lymphoedema are features of rosacea that seldom respond well to treatment. Rhinophyma is resistant to medical therapy but is simply managed by plastic surgery. Of the various manifestations of rosacea telangiectasia is the least amenable to improvement and additional camouflage advice may be valuable.

Perioral dermatitis

Perioral dermatitis is probably a variant of rosacea (Fig. 5.24). The disease is far commoner in women than men and the main aetiological feature appears to be the application of a topical steroid to a minor skin disorder such as acne or seborrhoeic eczema. Erythematous scaly patches and papules develop around the mouth and nose, or occasionally around the eye. Perioral dermatitis responds well to oxytetracycline 250 mg twice daily for 6−8 weeks, and relapses are uncommon if no further steroid is applied.

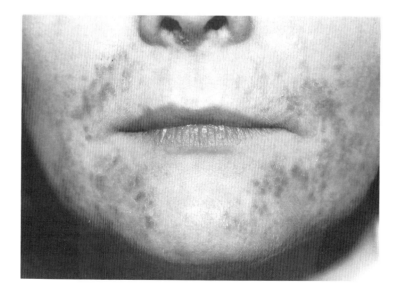

Fig. 5.24 Perioral dermatitis

Discoid lupus erythematosus (DLE)

The inflammatory plaques of discoid lupus erythematosus must be differentiated from rosacea (Fig. 5.25). DLE classically produces patches of erythema, scaling and telangiectasia on exposed sites like the face, scalp and ears. There is often an element of photosensitivity and sunscreens are an important part of treatment. DLE does not commonly progress to the systemic form of the disease but patients should be referred for biopsy and immunological assessment.

Most patients benefit from a topical steroid although initially a high potency preparation, such as betamethasone ointment, will be required. ROC Total Sunblock or Spectraban would be

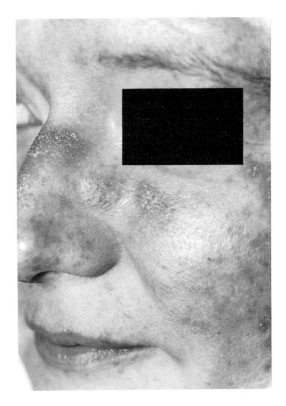

Fig. 5.25 Lupus erythematosus showing follicular plugging

suitable sunscreens. Resistant and extensive DLE will often require a systemic agent. The antimalarial drug chloroquine is used orally in a dose of 200 mg twice daily for 3–6 months.

Practice points

1 *Do not use topical steroids in rosacea. These are always contraindicated and ultimately will produce severe exacerbations ('steroid face').*
2 *DLE produces patches of erythema, scaling and telangiectasia on exposed sites like the face, scalp and ears.*

Scabies and other infestations

Scabies

Scabies is an infestation with the mite *Sarcoptes scabeii*. Spread of the disease occurs following skin contact of 30 minutes or so. The disease may be passed on during sexual activity but this is certainly not essential. Mothers transmit infection to babies and siblings transmit to each other.

Pruritus, the classical symptom of the condition, begins about 6 weeks after infection and is particularly troublesome at night when the body is warm. Burrows or vesicles identify the location of each mite (see Plate 8). In adults the wrists and finger webs are commonly involved. Adult males develop penile nodules. In infants scabies burrows and superficial pustules are easily seen on the soles of the feet. Axillary nodules may also be present in this age group. Secondary bacterial infection may occur which obscures the primary diagnosis (see Plate 9). To confirm the diagnosis the mite or eggs should be extracted from a burrow and examined under the low power microscope.

The diagnosis of scabies should be considered in all itching patients. Apart from atopic eczema it is the only disease likely to cause simultaneous itching in several members of a family. Infestation with *Sarcoptes scabeii* is common in the white and Asian communities but Afro-Caribbean individuals may be less susceptible. The development of severe and intractable itching associated with scaling and burrows on the finger webs, wrists, penis and other sites really should be, but often is not instantly diagnostic.

Once the diagnosis has been reached it is important that all members of the family and their intimate contacts, whether clinically affected or not, receive simultaneous treatment. In adults it is necessary to treat the entire surface of the body below the neck. Patients must be instructed to include such sites as the breasts, axillae, toes, finger webs and genitalia and not merely anoint the itching areas, which is useless. In children under two the head and neck must be included. After 24 hours (infants, 8 hours) the patient should have an ordinary bath with a change of personal and bed-linen. The soiled linen should be laundered in the ordinary way; no sterilization procedures are required. Even when treatment is completed successfully the itching will take 10-14 days to subside. Patients must be warned of this or they may continue to use the insecticide and develop an irritant dermatitis. Some patients in any case develop a post-scabies itch, without evidence of active infection. This phenomenon is particularly common in atopics and usually responds to treatment with hydrocortisone 1% cream.

A single application of 1% lindane cream or lotion (Lorexane: ICI; Quellada: Stafford-Miller) is normally required although some dermatologists recommend a second treatment one week after the first. Aqueous malathion 0.5% (Derbac-M: International Labs) is the latest insecticide to be employed in this disease and may be preferred in infants and during pregnancy.

Scabies is often associated with adolescents and young adults but in fact it is common in the elderly. Most dermatologists are familiar with outbreaks in rest homes and long-stay geriatric hospitals. Such outbreaks, which may affect many staff and patients, usually originate from one heavily infested individual who is thought to have eczema, psoriasis or any skin condition except scabies. Such individuals should be isolated until non-infectious and treatment should be given to the unit's other patients, and also staff and the relatives of staff. The immediate environment of heavily infested individuals, like those with crusted or 'Norwegian' scabies, can be heavily contaminated with mites and eggs. In the UK local authority environmental health departments will advise on the spraying of premises with a suitable insecticide such as malathion.

Practice points

1 *In scabies treat the whole family; treat the whole patient.*
2 *To ensure maximum compliance give patients a written instruction sheet (an example is given in the Appendix 1).*
3 *If the diagnosis is correct failures will be due to faulty technique, or an undetected contact.*

Pediculosis capitis

Infestation with the grey-brown head-louse, *Pediculus humanus*, is transmitted by hair contact. It predominantly affects children and females, with infections in adult males being less common. It should be considered as the most likely cause of an itchy scalp in childhood but non-itching adult victims can be found in head-louse epidemics and may be a source of re-infection. The presence of easily identifiable empty egg cases, or 'nits', should make the diagnosis simple. The nape of the neck and the hair behind the ears should be inspected.

Malathion 0.5% (Suleo-M: International Labs; Prioderm: Napp) or Carbaryl 0.5% (Suleo-C: International Labs; Carylderm: Napp) are highly effective. The agents are alternated to reduce the possibility of louse resistance developing. In the UK local pharmacists will be aware of the agent currently being employed in any area. The treatment (which is lethal to lice and eggs) can be repeated after 7 days for absolute certainty. Dead lice may continue to be shed from the hair for a day or two after treatment. The nits, though sterile, need to be removed by fine-tooth combing. Ordinary combing twice daily is believed to kill lice by breaking their legs. Insecticide containing shampoos are available but these are much less effective and cannot be recommended.

Pediculosis pubis

This represents infection with the crab-louse, *Pthirus pubis*. The brown lice, blue skin macules and eggs stuck to the pubic hair should make these unwelcome visitors easily recognized. The crab-louse is perfectly at home in any hairy area, provided that the hairs are not too dense. Check axillary hair, body hair, eyelashes and even scalp margins in affected individuals.

Aqueous malathion 0.5% lotion (Derbac-M) is now the preferred treatment. This preparation can be also applied with a cotton bud to the eyelashes if they are involved.

Arthropod bites and stings

Arthropods, such as mosquitoes, fleas and bed-bugs, bite in order to extract blood from the host. The characteristic wheal and punctum makes an ordinary bite easy to recognize. The very severity of bullous bites may obscure the diagnosis. All these changes seem to be the result of hypersensitivity of the host to antigens present in the creature's saliva.

In children excoriated and persistent flea-bites (papular urticaria) are commonly seen. The legs and other exposed sites are normally involved. Little clusters of 2 or 3 bites are characteristic. Almost all pets can carry insects that can cause this condition; the cat flea, *Ctenocephaloides felis* is the most troublesome. Not only may the animal itself habour fleas but bedding and favourite 'sleeping-spots' may contain eggs and larval stages. It is certainly not sufficient to treat any infected animal. Flea eggs may remain viable for up to twelve months after the original host has departed. Bedding should be washed in hot water and potential sites of infestation sprayed with an appropriate insecticide.

Among other troublesome species is the dog fur-mite, *Cheyletiella yasguri*. This creature bites the chest and abdomen of proud dog owners who hold or cuddle their pets. *Cheyletiella yasguri* can bite through clothing and produces monomorphic itchy red papular lesions. The bed-bug, *Cimex lectularis*, is active shortly before dawn; its bites are often bullous. When patients are bitten identification of the insect and avoidance are the only long-term solution. An antihistamine orally and hydrocortisone 1% cream may alleviate symptoms.

The stings of bees, wasps, hornets and the like are a defence mechanism. Hornet venom, for example, contains acetylcholine, peptides, histamine and other vaso-active amines; again hypersensitivity may account for much of the damage to the victim. After injection of venom local reactions can be quite severe and rarely angioedema or anaphylaxis may result. Most stings resolve spontaneously but severe local reactions may occasionally justify treatment with systemic antihistamines and topical steroids. In patients with a history of anaphylaxis it may be worth identifying the nature of the assailant by looking for venom specific IgE in the serum. In the UK desensitizing vaccines are available for those who have experienced life-threatening reactions but it is not universally agreed that desensitization is beneficial.

Practice points

1 *A biting insect cannot be identified by inspection of the bite.*
2 *If insect bites are suspected it may be more valuable to examine the pet than the patient.*

Tropical dermatology

Several tropical skin diseases are seen occasionally in UK hospital dermatology departments.

Leishmaniasis

Leishmaniasis, in the form of 'oriental sore', is common in the middle-east and Pakistan. The causative agent is *Leishmania tropica* transmitted by the bite of the sandfly. Affected patients develop scaly, fibrotic or ulcerated plaques on exposed skin. Self-healing with residual scarring is usual although patients with incomplete resistance may develop the chronic leishmania recidivans. Skin biopsy is diagnostic. The majority of patients require no active treatment at all but those that do respond to intra-muscular sodium stibogluconate. Surgical excision, and cryotherapy have also been used to treat cutaneous leishmaniasis.

Leprosy

Leprosy, especially new untreated cases of leprosy, is much less common. Patients with a high degree of resistance to *Mycobacterium leprae* develop the tuberculoid form of the disease which consists of a small number of hypopigmented anaesthetic patches often associated with peripheral nerve enlargement (see Plate 10). Such patients are diagnosed readily. Individuals with poor resistance develop the lepromatous form of the disease. This is associated with multiple cutaneous nodules, papules and plaques or simply skin thickening which is especially noticeable on the face. The skin lesions in lepromatous leprosy teem with mycobacteria.

General Practitioners should refer suspected cases to hospital for skin biopsy. It is never too early to start reassuring victims of this disease that treatment with modern drugs such as Dapsone, Rifampicin, and Clofazimine is highly effective although management of leprosy reaction neuropathy and some of the late complications can be quite testing. There has not been a case of leprosy being transmitted within the UK this century. Despite reassurance contacts in this country may sometimes manifest anxiety verging on hysteria.

Cutaneous larva migrans

Creeping eruption or cutaneous larva migrans resembles an itchy, erythematous thread under the skin and is caused by the larval stage of an animal hookworm (e.g. *Ankylostoma* spp.). These most unwelcome visitors are normally acquired by walking barefoot on infected soil or beaches in the West Indies, South America or tropical Africa. Thiabendazole ointment applied daily for 5 days is the treatment of choice for patients with only a few lesions.

Mycetoma

Injury to the foot, with subsequent sub-cutaneous fungal infection, is responsible for the development of mycetoma or Madura foot. The affected foot enlarges and subcutaneous nodules with multiple discharging sinuses develop. Various combinations of antifungal agents may be helpful but involvement of the underlying bone may necessitate amputation.

Tungiasis

Tungiasis is the infestation of the skin with the flea *Tunga penetrans*. It is prevalent in tropical Africa and also South America, the Caribbean and the west coast of the Indian subcontinent. Local names include jiggers and chigo. The female of the species burrows into the skin of an animal or human being and becomes engorged with blood and developing eggs. The typical skin lesion, usually seen on the toe or foot, is a pale pea-sized nodule with central black dot produced by the flea's abdominal segments. The nodules should be excised and an antibiotic cream applied. Affected individuals should be immunized against tetanus.

Benign and malignant skin tumours

Keloids

Keloids represent excessive and inappropriate fibroblastic response to skin damage. They are often precipitated by injury although this may be very slight. Distinction is usually drawn between hypertrophic scars, in which the firm, thickened and red tissue still confirms to the dimensions of the original injury, and true keloids where the masses of abnormal tissue are often rounded, painful and greatly exceed the dimensions of the original wound.

It is not clear why some individuals are particularly prone to keloid formation. It is commonest in Afro-Caribbean patients but can affect any ethnic group. The chest and upper arm are most frequently involved. It is better not to perform minor surgery in sites of predilection if this can possibly be avoided. Hypertrophic scars or small keloids often improve if injected with intralesional triamcinolone, although in black patients there is a risk of inducing perilesional hypopigmentation. Small keloids may benefit from having a steroid containing tape (Haelan Tape: Dista) applied to the area nightly.

Keratinous cysts

The name 'sebaceous cyst' is applied to the familiar firm mobile nodule often seen in middle-aged adults. This designation is not strictly correct since the cheesey contents of such cysts derives from keratin not sebum. Keratinous cysts are frequently found on the face, scalp, neck, shoulders and scrotum. The microscopic structure of the cyst wall resembles either normal epidermis (epidermoid cyst) or a hair shaft (pilar cyst). The cysts are easily excised under local anaesthetic.

Milia

Milia are small white or yellowish cysts containing keratin. They are usually most noticeable on the face and are most common in infants and adolescents. In infancy spontaneous resolution is usual. In older patients the overlying epidermis can be incised, and the contents of the cyst expressed, with a fine sterile needle.

Melanocytic naevi

Melanocytic (naevus cell) naevi are commonly called 'moles'. They can be divided into junctional, intradermal or compound naevi depending on the location of the majority of the naevus cells. Melanocytic naevi are seldom present at birth; the majority appear during childhood and become more numerous at adolescence. In the so-called Sutton's or 'halo' naevus a pigmented mole or moles become surrounded by a depigmented circle. This striking immunological phenomenon is usually seen in children or young adults particularly on the back and chest. It is *not* a sign of malignancy. Disappearance of the mole with repigmentation of the halo usually occurs spontaneously in a year or two.

The decision to excise an ordinary melanocytic naevus can be taken on purely cosmetic grounds. The chance of malignant transformation in a melanocytic naevus is very slight but any change in size or colour, bleeding or the development of itching justifies immediate excision biopsy.

Benign vascular tumours

Spider naevi are commonly seen on the face in children and young adults. They consist of a papule formed by a central arteriole with radiating peripheral vessels. Pregnancy and hepatic cirrhosis can predispose to their appearance but spider naevi usually arise spontaneously. Spiders are readily treated with a variety of minor destructive procedures such as lightly touching the central arteriole with a battery powered cautery or painting the entire lesion with trichloracetic acid.

The pyogenic granuloma is of course neither pyogenic nor granulomatous. They are benign acquired haemangiomas which normally develop in a previously traumatised area. Bleeding from the rather friable lesions can be alarming but is easily controlled with pressure. Curettage and cautery under local anaesthesia is the treatment of choice; relapse is rare. Beware of small lesions resembling pyogenic granulomas around the point of the chin, or indeed anywhere along the lower jaw. These may be abscesses tracking from periodontal infection. X-ray will show loss of alveolar bone around the affected tooth and an early dental opinion is required.

Juvenile melanomas can mimic a vascular lesion quite closely and form reddish nodules, 0.5-1 cm in size. They are benign naevi and are most frequently seen on the face in childhood. They have no malignant potential.

Seborrhoeic warts and skin tags

Seborrhoeic warts have no connection with sebum or sebaceous glands. The name derives from the somewhat greasy appearance of the surface of these superficial cauliflower-like lesions. They are correctly called basal cell papillomas and represent a benign epidermal tumour which is the almost invariable accompaniment of aging. Basal cell papillomas can be single or, more usually, multiple. They most commonly develop on the trunk; early lesions are flat and tan in colour but they become darker and more papillomatous with time. It is usually unnecessary to excise these tumours; removal by curettage and cautery is more convenient. Multiple basal cell papillomas can also be destroyed by cryotherapy.

Dermatosis papulosa nigra is the name given to the multiple flat pigmented lesions that develop on the faces of middle-aged and elderly Afro-Caribbean people. Histologically they resemble basal cell papillomas.

Skin tags are also common in the middle-aged and elderly of both sexes. They are most frequently located on the neck or axillae but can occur at any site. The lesions consist of a fibrovascular core covered in epidermis which can easily be snipped off with scissors under local anaesthesia.

Dermatofibromas

These are firm, smooth, button-like, pink or brown dermal nodules. They can occur anywhere but are commoner on the limbs than the trunk or face. Dermatofibromas are benign and are thought to be a reaction to dermal inflammation or insect bites. They seem to be more frequent in women than men and are treated by excision.

Skin malignancies

Skin malignancies are common; one in particular, the basal cell carcinoma, is the commonest of all human cancers (Table 5.9).

Malignant melanoma

Malignant melanoma is the most dangerous variety of skin cancer but ultimate prognosis can be greatly improved by

Table 5.9

Primary tumours	Malignant melanoma
	Non-melanoma epidermal tumours
	Basal cell carcinoma
	Squamous cell carcinoma
	Lymphoma
Pre-malignancies	Solar keratoses
	Bowen's disease
	Keratoacanthoma
Secondary tumours	e.g. breast, bronchus, lymphoma

early recognition and treatment. At least 1000 people die of the tumour in the UK every year; many malignant melanomas could be recognized and treated at an early stage if the public could be educated in self-examination (Table 5.10).

Malignant melanoma can arise from a pre-existing naevus or occur *de novo* (Table 5.11). Tumours are frequently deeply pigmented but this is not universal; truly amelanotic lesions occasionally occur.

Lentigo maligna is the least aggressive variety (Fig. 5.26). This characteristically presents as a pigmented macule on the face of an elderly individual with a history of excessive sun

Table 5.10   Suspicious signs in pigmented skin tumours

Recent change of shape
Diameter of >0.5 cm
Recent change of colour; pigment variability
Itching
Bleeding
Irregularity of tumour edge

Table 5.11   Patterns of malignant melanoma

Lentigo maligna
Superficial spreading
Nodular
Acral

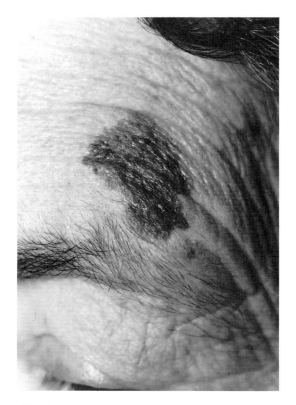

Fig. 5.26 Hutchinson's lentigo maligna melanoma

exposure. Lentigo maligna can be regarded as malignant melanoma *in situ*, but a true invasive melanoma may develop after some years. If adequately excised the prognosis is excellent but some clinicians favour a less mutilating approach such as cryotherapy.

Superficial spreading melanomas are thin lesions with only a limited propensity to invade. Patients will usually give a history of a pigmented macule that is changing shape or colour. Itching or the 'sticking' of a lesion to clothing are suspicious signs. The pigmentation of a melanoma is normally not homogenous and irregularity of the surface or margin is worrying. Nodular melanoma is the most aggressive variant and may grow rapidly (Fig. 5.27). It is widely believed that some

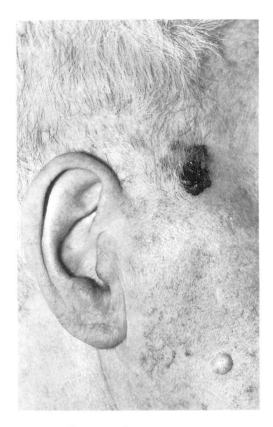

Fig. 5.27 Nodular malignant melanoma

nodular melanomas evolve from superficial spreading melanomas by entering a phase of vertical growth. The acral lentiginous melanoma is rare in whites. It occurs on the palms, soles, and nail-beds.

There does appear to be a relationship between sun exposure and the development of melanomas. It seems that short-term excessive exposure can initiate the tumour in a susceptible individual. The frequency of the tumour is increasing world wide among white populations and malignant melanoma is the one tumour commoner in the more affluent members of society.

The primary treatment of melanoma is excision and grafting.

A 5 cm clear margin is desirable round a nodular melanoma. The optimal resection margin round a superficial spreading melanoma is still a matter of debate but a 1 cm margin is probably sufficient for lesions less than 1 mm in thickness. Naturally the management of this tumour is usually the province of plastic surgery. The response of secondary melanoma deposits to any regime of radiotherapy or chemotherapy is very poor and this places great responsibility on those who diagnose and treat primary lesions.

Basal cell carcinoma (BCC)

The BCC or rodent ulcer usually develops on the central face and is seen in the middle-aged and elderly (Fig. 5.28). The BCC, like other non-melanoma skin cancers, is closely linked to accumulated actinic exposure. Consequently it is seen earlier in white skinned individuals living in areas with a high level of sunshine. Classically BCCs have a raised pearly edge, central ulceration and prominent overlying

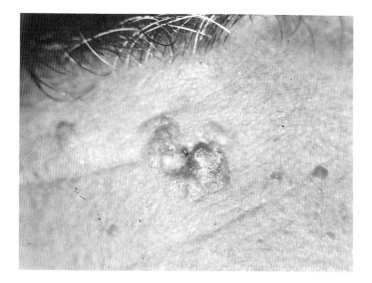

Fig. 5.28 Basal cell carcinoma

telangiectasia. Pigmented or morphoeic forms may produce diagnostic difficulties.

BCCs do not metastasize although neglected tumours can produce marked local destruction. Curettage and cautery is a widely used method of destroying small tumours but does not permit histological assessment of the adequacy of treatment. Formal surgical excision overcomes this disadvantage and is the method of choice for areas such as the eyelid and naso-labial fold where damaging extension of the tumour into deep structures can occur at an early stage.

Squamous cell carcinoma (SCC)

This tumour also usually occur on light exposed areas such as the face, ear and the hands. They can develop as an occupa-tional skin problem in individuals who have had regular con-tact with tars or oils. They normally present as solitary nodular, ulcerated or hyperkeratotic lesions. SCCs grow more rapidly than BCCs and show a greater propensity to metasta-size. Excision is the treatment of choice.

Solar keratoses and Bowen's disease

Solar keratoses are small, scaly, erythematous lesions which occur on light exposed sites such as the ears, face, backs of hands, and the bald scalp. They are pre-malignant and may occasionally evolve into SCCs. Bowen's disease represents carcinoma *in situ* and presents as a well demarcated scaly, erythematous plaque which is often confused with a solitary patch of eczema or psoriasis. Lesions can be destroyed by surgery, cryotherapy or with topical 5% 5-Fluorouracil (Efudix: Roche).

Keratoacanthoma

Histologically a keratoacanthoma closely resembles a SCC but does not invade the dermis. This tumour grows very rapidly and can reach full size in 2−4 weeks. There is a prominent raised edge with a central keratin plug. Ultimately spontaneous involution occurs but early surgical excision produces a better final cosmetic result. Keratoacanthomas can be effectively treated by curettage. Unfortunately a histopathologist finds it difficult to distinguish between a keratoacanthoma and an invasive SCC unless the specimen includes the 'shoulder' and the centre of the lesion. For this reason excision biopsy is preferred.

Cutaneous T-cell lymphoma

This disorder was previously known as mycosis fungoides and is the primary skin lymphoma (Fig. 5.29). The natural history of the disease is very long, often extending over several decades.

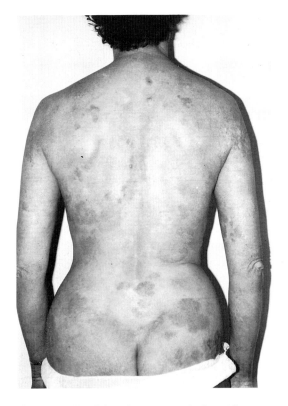

Fig. 5.29 Cutaneous T-cell lymphoma (mycosis fungoides)

Irregular erythematous and pigmented plaques develop which very gradually show signs of infiltration. Cutaneous nodules and ulcers form in late stages of the disease and clinical lymph-node enlargement is also delayed.

For many years the manifestations of this disorder are controllable with topical steroids and PUVA therapy. In the UK treatment with chemotherapy or radiotherapy is confined to patients with some evidence of extra-cutaneous spread and the response of the disease to these types of treatment is often unsatisfactory.

Secondary deposits

It is relatively rare to see patients presenting to a dermatologist with metastatic cancer (Table 5.12).

Table 5.12 Common tumours associated with skin metastases

Male	Female
Lung	Breast
Colon	Colon
Melanoma	Melanoma
Kidney	Ovary
Lymphoma	Lymphoma

Bronchial carcinoma and adenocarcinoma of the kidney may present with skin secondaries. Secondary breast cancer never presents before the primary disease although Paget's disease of the nipple may lead to the discovery of an intraductal carcinoma.

Non-metastatic manifestations of internal malignancy

Abdominal tumours may be associated with velvety pigmented plaques in the flexures called acanthosis nigricans (Fig. 5.30). Carcinoma of the bronchus and ovary have been linked to annular or gyrate erythematous skin lesions (erythema annulare centrifugum). Aquired ichthyosis may develop in sufferers

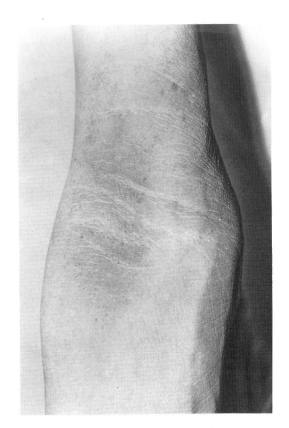

Fig. 5.30 Acanthosis nigricans; velvety flexural skin

from lymphoma. Generalized pruritus and dermatomyositis have both been described in association with tumours but often occur in individuals without malignant disease.

Practice points

1 *Solar keratoses, squamous cell carcinomas and basal cell carcinomas of the skin are common on light-exposed sites.*
2 *Do everything possible to encourage patients to report tumours that enlarge, itch, bleed or change colour.*

Leg ulcers

Ulceration of the lower leg is a major cause of discomfort and disability in the middle-aged and elderly. The majority of ulcers have a vascular origin. It has been estimated that at any one time there may be up to 100 000 patients in the UK suffering from vascular leg ulcers of whom 75% receive treatment in the community.

Venous ulcers

Sustained venous hypertension is the commonest cause of persistent ulceration of the leg (Fig. 5.31). The fundamental cause

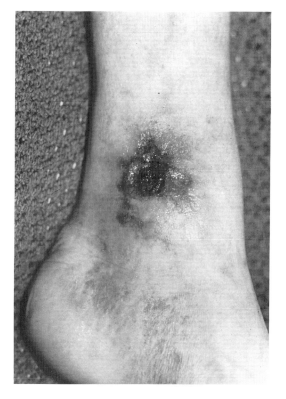

Fig. 5.31 Venous leg ulceration

of venous hypertension appears to lie in damage, often post-phlebitic, to valves in the perforating veins that communicate between the superficial and deep venous systems of the leg. Destruction of these valves results in the transmission of excessive pressure from the deep venous system into the superficial system. One contemporary theory holds that this pressure causes enlargement of the dermal capillary bed which leaks red cells and fibrinogen containing fluid. A fibrin cuff forms around small blood vessels which leads to impaired gaseous exchange and tissue anoxia. Minor trauma or infection are often the initiating events that finally precipitate ulceration of damaged skin.

Venous ulcers frequently form above and behind the malleoli of the ankle. The ulcers are irregular, superficial and relatively painless. Other signs of venous hypertension such as haemosiderin pigmentation, a venous flare, oedema or venous eczema are often visible. Varicosity of the leg veins are of little significance.

The physical removal of devitalized tissue, slough and debris, with scissors and forceps is an essential preliminary to the formation of healthy granulation tissue. Subsequently the reduction of oedema and the provision of adequate support is of far more importance to the subsequent healing of venous ulcers than the application of antibacterial substances. Although plentiful bacteria are found on the surface of ulcers their pathogenic role has been greatly exaggerated (Table 5.13).

Table 5.13   Antiseptics used in leg ulcer treatment

0.05% chlorhexidine gluconate (Hibitane: ICI)
Hydrogen peroxide (Hioxyl: Quinoderm)
Povidone-iodine (Betadine: Napp)

Venous ulcers are commonly associated with patches of venous eczema, or medicament induced contact dermatitis, to which such patients are particularly prone. Preparations containing sensitizers such as parabens, chlorocresol and lanolin are often difficult to avoid. Ulcer therapists must be alert to the development of itching, erythema and vesiculation that could indicate a medicament allergy. Topical corticosteroid preparations are very helpful in the control of eczema but the weakest possible preparation should be employed, for preference hydrocortisone ointment, and the steroid should be kept out of the ulcer itself.

External pressure retards the development of oedema and reverses the flow of blood from the deep venous plexuses through incompetent perforators. The method chosen should be cosmetically acceptable and permit the use of ordinary footware. Support bandaging is still widely used. In this technique a piece of plain paraffin gauze is cut to size and placed on the ulcer followed by a pad of gauze material which soaks up some exudate and more evenly distributes the pressure from the overlying bandage. Next a medicated paste bandage is applied such as Zincaband (Seton) or Viscopaste PB7 (Smith & Nephew). These consist of zinc oxide, starch and glycerine spread on a bleached cotton strip 6 m × 3.5 cm. Strips of the bandage are applied from the tarso-metatarsal junction to the tibial tuberosity. It is important to obtain a 'smooth' finish without any folds or tucks which might cause pressure necrosis of the underlying skin.

The last step in the procedure is the application of the compression bandage itself. Common examples of these are Poroplast (Scholl), and Secure Forte (Johnson & Johnson). The compression bandage covers the paste bandage strips completely. The pressure exerted is partly determined by the materials from which the bandage is fabricated and partly by the tension applied. During application it is important to maintain an even 'pull'. The patient should feel that the completed dressing is firm but not tight. There is no virtue in changing this type of dressing frequently; a healing ulcer should be interfered with as little as possible. Reapplication is required when the bandage becomes soaked with exudate, and malodorous; once or twice weekly is usually sufficient.

Elastic compression stockings are perhaps the most common treatment of all for chronic venous insufficiency. A variety of materials, patterns and sizes are available and a simple illustrated guide for UK prescribers is to be found in the 'Dressings, Hosiery and Appliances' section of the *Monthly Index of Medical Specialties*. (Medical Mailing Co., P.O. Box 60, Loughborough LE11 OWP). One example of the stockings available is shown in Table 5.14.

Prescribers should specify the quantity, compression class, length and brand-name required. Calf-length compression stockings are quite adequate for the management of venous ulceration. They should be applied before rising in the morning and worn all day.

Table 5.14 Elastic compression stockings for chronic venous insufficiency

Class	Compression (mmHg)	Make	Model	Fittings	Indication
1	18–25	Sigvaris	601	Calf	Mild varicosis, oedema
2	27–35	Sigvaris	902	Calf, thigh	Mild venous insufficiency
		Sigvaris	503	Calf, thigh, tights	
3	36–48	Sigvaris	504	Calf, thigh	Oedema, ulcers

NEW LEG ULCER TREATMENTS

Absorbent carbohydrate polymers are now widely available. These are formulated into powders consisting of inert, spherical microbeads. When applied to ulcers these preparations absorb exudate and remove particulate material. The first of these products to be marketed in the UK was dextranomer (Debrisan: Pharmacia); one system simultaneously releases iodine as it absorbs (Iodosorb: Perstop). In general the ulcers should be cleaned and covered with a layer of polymer 3–4 mm thick. The area should be covered by a dry dressing, and a removable compression stocking or equivalent applied. When the dressing is changed the old material can be washed off with water or saline. Polymer powders are not really suitable for dry wounds. After application to wet wounds they are removed before they become saturated. In practice this involves daily or twice daily application.

The occlusive hydrocolloids seem to be an important advance. An example is Granuflex (Convatec). Granuflex is a sheet with an adhesive inner face and an outer surface of impervious polyurethane foam. The hydrocolloid contains gelatin, pectin and carboxy-methylcellulose. Once applied the exudate from the wound is absorbed to produce a gel which fills the space between the ulcer surface and the dressing. The gel creates a good, moist healing environment but also possesses a penetrating and unpleasant odour. This is normally a problem only if the dressing leaks. Dressing removal is easy and painless.

ANTIBIOTICS

Although frequently used antibiotics have really only a very limited role in treatment, since it is quite impractical, and indeed unnecessary, to think of 'sterilizing' ulcers. Spreading streptococcal cellulitis (erysipelas) can originate from a leg ulcer. This disease is potentially very destructive and should be vigorously treated with penicillin. Ulcers which are highly purulent and offensive may be infected with gram-negative anaerobic organisms such as bacteroides. A 2 week course of metronidazole may improve this distressing symptom.

ULCER PREVENTION

Once a venous ulcer has healed signs of chronic venous insufficiency will almost invariably be present. These include dilated subcutaneous veins, pigmentation, and scarring. A combination of induration and atrophie blanche is sometimes called liposclerosis. Patients showing these features should adopt an ulcer prevention regime by:
- Taking daily exercise
- Performing daily postural drainage to minimise oedema
- Avoiding the minor trauma that precipitates ulceration
- Wearing elastic support stockings or tights
  Oedema and the other symptoms of venous hypertension

may be improved by the use of oxerutins (Paroven: Zyma). This drug reduces abnormal leakage from the capillaries. In several studies the use of stanozolol (Stromba: Sterling) combined with elastic stockings has been shown to improve liposclerosis and the symptoms of venous disease, although it is not certain that the rate of ulcer healing is improved.

Ischaemic ulcers

Arterial ulcers are painful. Typically the patients complain that the discomfort is worst at night when the limb is elevated in bed. The ulcers are 'punched-out' and frequently contain a thick necrotic slough. Any area on the leg or foot can be involved but the dorsum of the foot, heel or anterior tibial areas are common locations. Small painful ulcers on the medial border of the great toe are classically the result of defective arterial perfusion. There will normally be other signs of ischaemia such as thickening of nails and absent foot pulses. Atheroma is the commonest cause of peripheral vascular disease. Cigarette smoking is widely believed to be an associated cause in many patients. Beta-blockers and, less commonly, ergot alkaloids may cause further deterioration.

The management of ischaemic ulcers is always difficult and the prognosis, particularly in the elderly, is dismal. Regular cleansing and debridement of the ulcer should be arranged. Topical antiseptics, hydrogen peroxide cream, and polymer powders have all been used although the benefits of local treatment are minimal. The material selected should be held in place by the lightest possible dressing. It cannot be stressed too strongly that the use of external support is contra-indicated since this can further prejudice an already compromised cutaneous circulation.

It is essential that adequate analgesia is provided, although not infrequently this is impossible to achieve without resorting to opiates. The role of other drugs in the management of established ulceration is controversial. Conventional vasodilators, though widely used, are almost certainly ineffective. Naftidrofuryl (Praxilene: Lipha) has been extensively used in peripheral vascular disease. It is an antispasmodic that also has a direct effect on cellular metabolism which improves the function of ischaemic cells at reduced oxygen levels. Oxpentifylline (Trental: Hoechst) is a rheologically active agent which should improve the blood flow through the microcirculation. Despite these theoretical considerations neither drug has proved especially beneficial when given orally. In hospital intravenous infusion of either drug can produce quite impressive, if temporary, improvement.

The only definitive treatment for ischaemic limbs is surgical reconstruction of the major leg arteries. However by no means all types of blockage are amenable to correction. Lumbar sympathectomy can be performed surgically or by phenol injection. Sympathectomy should abolish intrinsic smooth muscle tone in cutaneous arterioles thus improving skin blood flow. This procedure may improve limb perfusion but ablative surgery should not be delayed too long if pain is intractable and the limb is clearly not salvable.

Practice points

1 *External support is the most important factor in the healing of venous ulcers but is harmful in the presence of ischaemia.*
2 *Squamous cell carcinomas and basal cell carcinomas can complicate long-standing ulceration of any cause.*
3 *Patients with ischaemic leg ulcers should be referred to a vascular surgeon.*

Urticaria

Urticaria is a vascular reaction pattern resulting in transient whealing of the skin, sometimes accompanied by oedematous swellings of the subcutaneous tissues (Fig. 5.32). The disease is of variable severity and is common in all age groups, especially children and young adults. Itching may be severe. The common name for the condition is 'nettle-rash' or 'hives'.

Urticaria can be chronic although individual erythematous wheals are transient, lasting for only a few hours. The rash often shows diurnal variation and may be associated with angioedema of the eyes, lips and other sites (Fig. 5.33). The

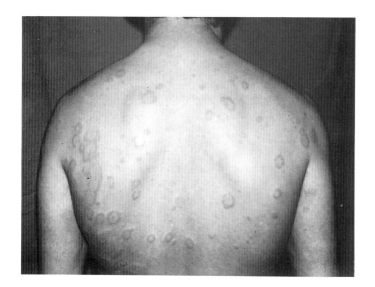

Fig. 5.32 Urticaria

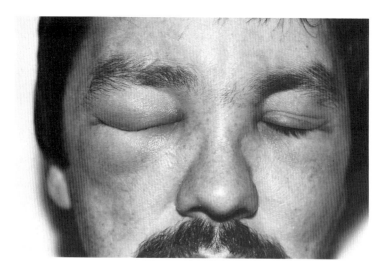

Fig. 5.33 Angioedema of the face

diagnosis is usually easy to make but occasionally angioedema of, say, the face needs to be carefully distinguished from an acute contact dermatitis. A dermatitis is more persistent and will exhibit features of epidermal involvement such as scaling and vesiculation.

Some types of urticaria occur spontaneously; others are precipitated by physical stimuli such as cold, heat, sunlight or light pressure (dermographism). 'Cholinergic' urticaria consists of multiple tiny wheals with a surrounding erythematous flare. The problem is usually seen on the trunk of adolescents and is associated with sweating. Exercise, hot baths or even spicy food can trigger off an attack. In all patterns the basic mechanism appears to be release of histamine, kinins, prostaglandins and vaso-active amines from degranulating mast cells.

No laboratory test will confirm the diagnosis of urticaria nor distinguish between immunologically and non-immunologically induced types. In 75% of patients with chronic urticaria no conclusive cause is discovered. Rarely urticaria is linked with a systemic illness but I must stress that the majority of patients are fit children and young adults (Table 5.15). The small likelyhood of obtaining positive results means that investigation should be restricted to severe and unresponsive cases.

Table 5.15   Medical problems associated with urticaria

Infections, e.g. hepatitis
Neoplasms
Thyrotoxicosis
Connective tissue disorders, e.g. SLE
Chronic candida infections
Gut infestation with protozoa or worms

Acute episodes of urticaria are commonly attributed to ingestion of foodstuffs. Milk, eggs, strawberries, nuts and shellfish are notorious in this respect. Codeine, salicylates and azo-dyes like tartrazine (E102) may exacerbate attacks.

Systemic antihistamines are the cornerstone of treatment

for urticaria. Because sleepiness is an unacceptable side-effect in most active patients the development of non-sedating drugs in the 1980s was a considerable advance e.g. astemizole 10 mg at night (Hismanal: Janssen) or terfenadine 60 mg twice daily (Triludan: Merrell Dow). The combination of a conventional antihistamine (H_1 blocker) with an H_2 blocker (e.g. ranitidine or cimetidine) may result in enhanced effectiveness. Sufferers from urticaria must appreciate the need for regular treatment. Several days treatment may be required before any effect is seen and I would normally continue treatment for 6 weeks before breaking off to see if spontaneous resolution has occurred.

The physical urticarias respond very poorly to antihistamines although hydroxyzine or cyproheptadine (Periactin: MSD) may be tried. Doxepin 10 mg 3 times daily (Sinequan: Pfizer) has the reputation of being helpful in cold urticaria. Every attempt should be made to teach the patients avoidance strategies. It is obviously essential for those with cold urticaria to avoid iced drinks and cold-water bathing. Dermographism is quite common in young adults but usually is not severe enough to require active treatment.

Systemic steroids have a limited place in the short-term management of very severe urticarial attacks but under these circumstances concurrent antihistamine treatment should also be started. Very rarely there may be universal urticaria, glottal or laryngeal oedema, and collapse. In these circumstances give 0.5 ml adrenaline 1:1000 intramuscularly, 200 mg hydrocortisone i.v., and promethazine 50 mg i.m. Emergency tracheostomy may be required if the airway is compromised. Acute episodes of this type usually follow severe reactions to serum or penicillin.

An uncommon form of angioedema is familial and dominantly inherited. Familial angioedema is associated with a deficiency of an inhibitor of a glycoprotein complement faction (C_1 esterase). Episodes of laryngeal and tracheal oedema may occur and infusions of fresh frozen plasma can prove life-saving if given early enough. Attacks of this rare condition can be prevented by maintenance treatment with danazol (Danol: Winthrop) or stanozolol (Stromba: Sterling).

Practice points

1 *The tendency of urticaria is towards gradual spontaneous improvement; play for time.*
2 *Do not abandon an antihistamine as ineffective until it has been used for a week at the maximum tolerated dose on a regular basis.*
3 *Do not prescribe regular antihistamines for children with urticaria unless pruritus is persistent and distressing.*

Skin diseases in general medicine

This section contains brief accounts of several skin complaints which are a secondary consequence of internal disease:
- pyoderma gangrenosum
- erythema nodosum
- necrobiosis lipoidica
- connective tissue diseases
- purpura and bruising
- inherited disorders
- AIDS

Pyoderma gangrenosum

Pyoderma gangrenosum is a destructive and rapidly progressing, ulcerative, inflammatory dermatosis. The disease may be idiopathic but perhaps half the affected patients have a systemic illness (Table 5.16).

Table 5.16 Diseases associated with pyoderma gangrenosum

Inflammatory bowel disease
Rheumatoid arthritis
Myelo-proliferative disorders
Paraproteinaemia
Chronic active hepatitis

Any area may be affected although the leg is the commonest location. A central necrotic ulcer is surrounded by

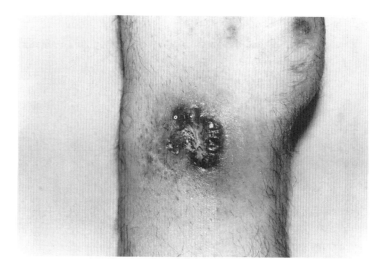

Fig. 5.34 Pyoderma gangrenosum

a swollen, cyanotic margin and an erythematous flare. There is little constitutional upset. Pyoderma gangrenosum (Fig. 5.34) can be very destructive but is usually responsive to high-dose systemic steroid therapy, although some patients will require 'steroid-sparing agents' like azathioprine.

Erythema nodosum

Erythema nodosum poses more of a diagnostic than a therapeutic challenge. Painful red nodules develop on the shins or less frequently the arms (see Plate 11). They fade over a 4–6 week period leaving residual bruising. Arthralgia may be prominent. The disease is commoner in females than males and the majority of the victims are young adults.

An antecedent cause for EN can usually be discovered and it is believed the pathogenesis involves immune-complex deposition in dermal blood vessels (Table 5.17). In the UK the majority of cases are associated with sarcoidosis or are post-streptococcal. In southern Europe yersinia enterocolitis is commonly responsible and in the USA coccidiomycosis or blastomycosis. EN leprosum lesions are a feature of leprosy reactions.

Most patients with arthralgia find aspirin or indomethacin

Table 5.17 Diseases associated with erythema nodosum

Streptococcal infection
Sarcoidosis
Tuberculosis
Inflammatory bowel disease
Drugs (sulphonamides, oral contraceptives)
Behets syndrome

helpful. The lesions themselves can be treated with potent topical steroids under support bandaging. Bed-rest is helpful in the most severe cases.

Patients in the UK should have a throat swab taken and a ASO titre checked. If there is a history of contact with open tuberculosis then EN plus a positive Mantoux reaction would be sufficient evidence on which to commence anti-tuberculous chemotherapy. If sarcoidosis is the cause of the EN then a chest X-ray will normally show bilateral hilar lymphadenopathy. Sarcoidosis may produce other types of skin involvement such as infiltrated scars, cutaneous nodules or an indurated plaque over the nose or cheek (lupus pernio).

Necrobiosis lipoidica

Skin problems associated with diabetes include staphylococcal and candida infections. Diabetic neuropathy can be associated with ulcers of the foot, and hyperlipidaemia with skin xanthomas. Necrobiosis lipoidica is usually seen on the shins (see Plate 12). The disorder is commoner in women than men with over half the affected patients being diabetic. It produces an asymptomatic, irregular, waxy, yellowish-red plaque with prominent blood vessels; ulceration may occur. Treatment is ineffective.

Connective tissue diseases

SYSTEMIC LUPUS ERYTHEMATOSUS (SLE)

SLE usually presents in young adults and shows female preponderance. SLE is a multi-system disorder but 80% patients have skin manifestations which include photosensitivity, alopecia, and facial lesions. Arthralgia, anaemia, and leucopenia are common. Renal and neuro-psychiatric manifestations are rarer but of major prognostic importance. On the basis of immunological investigations SLE has been extensively sub-divided but almost all patients have a positive test for antinuclear antibodies and the presence of anti-DNA antibodies is virtually specific for the disease. Systemic steroids are the corner-stone of treatment. Antimalarials and immunosuppressants are also widely used.

SYSTEMIC SCLEROSIS

Systemic sclerosis is also commoner in women. The disease produces a combination of vascular damage, fibrosis and immunological abnormalities. Clinical diagnosis is based on a triad of features:

1 *Raynaud's disease:* present in more than 90% patients.

2 *Skin manifestations:* including facial sclerosis, facial telangiectasia and pigmentary changes.

3 *Internal organ involvement:* most commonly arthralgia, oesophageal involvement and pulmonary fibrosis.

There is no curative treatment for systemic sclerosis but individual symptoms can be improved. Morphoea is possibly a localized variant of this disorder. An indurated violaceous patch develops which evolves into a firm plaque of hairless ivory coloured skin (see Plate 13). Morphoea can involve the face, trunk or limbs.

DERMATOMYOSITIS

Patients with dermatomyositis have evidence of a proximal myopathy together with a cluster of cutaneous features which include:
● periorbital erythema and oedema
● periungual telangiectasia
● lichenoid papules on the fingers (see Plate 14)
● psoriasiform plaques on the elbows
    In addition to the clinical features, the diagnosis is reached

on the basis of EMG findings, raised levels of creatine phosphokinase, or other muscle enzymes, and muscle biopsy. Treatment is with systemic steroids and immunosuppressants.

Purpura and bruising

These signs commonly lead to patient being referred to dermatologists, haematologists and physicians. Before investigating it is wise to establish that the bruising is spontaneous; do not be confused by traumatic bruising, or patients with scabies who scratch until they bruise. Steroids, scurvy and senility lead to bruising because of reduced soft-tissue support for capillaries. The bruising associated with Ehlers–Danlos syndrome probably has a similar origin.

If these causes are eliminated it is reasonable to perform a full blood count, biochemical profile, serum protein electrophoresis and coagulation studies (Table 5.18).

Table 5.18 Causes of purpura and bruising

Thrombocytopenia	Primary auto-immune	
	Secondary	Leukaemia, drugs
Coagulation disorders		
Dysproteinaemias	Paraproteinaemias	
	Hyperglobulinaemia	SLE, Sjögrens syndrome
Systemic diseases		Uraemia, liver disease

An immune complex vasculitis can produce purpura in addition to urticarial wheals, nodules and ulcers. An example is Henoch–Schönlein purpura which affects young children. This disorder, which may follow a streptococcal infection, results in arthralgia, abdominal pain, haematuria and an urticarial or purpuric rash on the buttocks and lower legs. Vasculitis can also be associated with drug rashes, SLE, and polyarteritis nodosa; many affected patients have no definable precipitating cause.

Inherited disorders

EHLERS-DANLOS SYNDROME (EDS)

EDS is a genetically determined disorder of connective tissue. At least eight distinct varieties are known with dominant, recessive and X-linked patterns of inheritance. It is believed that the fundamental cause of EDS are abnormalities in the structure of collagen and much time has been spent trying to ascertain the molecular basis of the syndrome. The variants of EDS share common features.

1 Major features: joint hypermobility and skin hyper-extensibility.

2 Minor features: bruising tendency, wide, 'cigarette-paper' scars, and skin 'pseudotumours'.

All types of EDS show a bleeding tendency and occasionally patients present with spontaneous rupture of an artery. The presence of any of the above features requires referral for expert assessment.

NEUROFIBROMATOSIS

This disorder is a dominantly inherited developmental abnormality of neural crest cell derivatives. The commoner peripheral form of the disease presents in infancy. Clinical features include café-au-lait macules, axillary freckling, cutaneous neurofibromas and kyphoscoliosis (Fig. 5.35). Individuals with the central form of neurofibromatosis develop bilateral acoustic neuromas or meningiomas in the second or third decade. Some cutaneous features are usually present.

PEUTZ-JEGHER'S SYNDROME

In this dominantly inherited syndrome multiple oval pigmented macules appear in and around the mouth. Secondary areas of involvement are around the nose and on the fingers. The importance of this finding is the associated adenomatous polyps found throughout the gastro-intestinal tract but especially in the jejunum and colon. The presence of the polyps

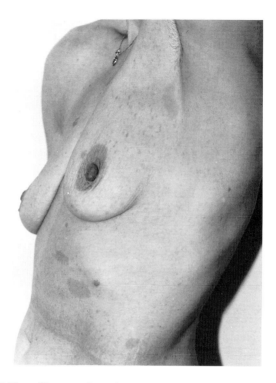

Fig. 5.35 Neurofibromatosis; café-au-lait macules

may lead to intussusception and a small percentage become malignant.

PSEUDOXANTHOMA ELASTICUM (PXE)

PXE is a disorder of elastic tissue which affects the skin, eyes and cardiovascular system. Doughy plaques of yellowish skin develop on the sides of the neck and also in areas like the axillae, antecubital and popliteal fossae. The rest of the skin is normal. Angeoid streaks are visible on retinoscopy. A portion of affected patients develop medial artery calcification or necrosis of the aorta and its major branches. This may lead to gastro-intestinal haemorrhage, claudication or angina.

Acquired immune deficiency syndrome (AIDS) and the skin

Infection with the human immunodeficiency virus 1, (HIV-1) has become a major public health problem during the last 10 years. There can be few doctors now unaware that there are several groups with a high risk of becoming infected with HIV. These include male homosexuals, the female partners of bisexual men, intravenous drug abusers, those recently resident in Haiti and, before blood product screening, haemophiliacs. At present in the UK the risk of sexual transmission to monogamous, even serially monogamous, heterosexuals is small but it is recognized that in the USA heterosexuals, and in particular intravenous drug abusers and their contacts, form the fastest growing group of AIDS patients.

Infection with HIV is associated with several clinical syndromes. These include:

1 Acute glandular fever-like illness.
2 Persistent generalized lymphadenopathy (PGL).
3 AIDS-related complex (ARC).
4 Symptomless carrier status.
5 AIDS.

In many cases infection with HIV may be unaccompanied by any symptoms and signs. Some patients will develop an acute glandular fever like illness in which lymphadenopathy is associated with an erythematous macular rash. This problem is self-limiting and probably occurs at the time of sero-conversion.

PGL represents multisite, unexplained, lymphadenopathy. This can be associated cutaneously with seborrhoeic dermatitis and severe herpes zoster. ARC is defined as symptomatic infection with HIV in the absence of opportunistic infection or tumour. Again seborrhoeic dermatitis has been described in this syndrome, as has oral candidiasis. The commonest presentation of established AIDS is *Pneumocystis carinii* pneumonia (60%). There is an overall diffuse pigmentation. The skin gives the appearance of having aged rapidly and the body is wasted.

OPPORTUNISTIC INFECTION

Ano-genital herpes simplex can be very severe with progressive ulceration. Facial molluscum contagiosum and severe
oral candidiasis are rare, but not unknown, in immunologically
normal adults and have both been frequently described in
AIDS patients. Extensive and unresponsive tinea cruris
or corporis have been described, as has severe scabies
infestation.

CUTANEOUS TUMOURS

Kaposi's sarcoma is a rare neoplasm of blood vessels often
appearing as purple, raised, non-tender skin nodules or plaques.
The palate may be involved. In AIDS patients the lesions are
usually multiple but may be solitary and can, in fact, closely
mimic other banal problems such as bruises or pyogenic granulomas. An early hospital referral for skin biopsy is desirable
in patients at risk. This tumour is not restricted to AIDS
patients although 25% of those infected may present in this
way. The 'classical' presentation of the disease was chocolate
brown, slowly progressive plaques on the legs of elderly individuals of Jewish or East European extraction. AIDS patients
have an increased risk of developing other tumours, in particular B-cell lymphomas. Involvement of extra-nodal sites, such
as skin, CNS, and gastro-intestinal tract is common.

SEBORRHOEIC DERMATITIS AND OTHER DERMATOSES

Seborrhoeic dermatitis is a common red, scaly rash affecting
the face and chest. There is a high prevalence in AIDS patients
who may develop a severe and explosive form of the disease.
In these individuals it is often associated with a facial folliculitis; a more extensive necrotizing folliculitis affecting forearms, back and thighs is also described.

HAIRY LEUKOPLAKIA OF THE MOUTH

White, warty lesions particularly along the lateral aspect of the tongue and also the buccal mucosa. This may be a viral infection but the exact aetiology is unknown.

Pregnancy and the skin

Physiological changes

Hyperpigmentation is extremely common during pregnancy, although least obvious in the fair-haired and fair skinned. The development of the linea nigra in the centre of the abdomen is well-known, as is the accentuation of normally pigmented areas such as the areolae and ano-genital region. Over 50% of pregnant women develop chloasma or 'mask of pregnancy'. This is a symmetrical irregular macular hyperpigmentation affecting the cheeks or the central facial area. All these types of pigmentation diminish after delivery but women seldom return completely to their pre-gravid state.

Stretch marks (striae gravidarum) are seen in most pregnant women during the last trimester. The abdomen, breasts, and thighs are commonly affected sites although severity is very variable. The incidence of the common acquired vascular naevus known as the spider angioma is much increased during pregnancy. Treatment should be avoided at this stage since most regress after delivery. Palmar erythema is a prominent finding in many pregnant patients as are vulval and leg varicosities. These vascular changes are thought to be related to high circulating oestrogen levels.

Many patients state that their hirsutism began, or deteriorated, during pregnancy. The upper lip and suprapubic midline hair seem particularly sensitive. This phenomenon is probably produced by a prolonged anagen stage induced by raised progesterone levels. The same explanation accounts for the apparent increase in the length and thickness of scalp hair during pregnancy. Immediately after delivery there is a rapid conversion of anagen to telogen follicles, with subsequent hair loss and diffuse alopecia (telogen effluvium).

Skin problems specific to pregnancy

POLYMORPHIC ERUPTION OF PREGNANCY (PEP)

This disorder is also known as toxic erythema of pregnancy but is not related to pre-eclamptic toxaemia. PEP is most commonly seen in primagravidae. It usually develops in the last 2 or 3 weeks of pregnancy although it can occur at any time in the second or third trimester. Urticated erythematous plaques or 'iris' lesions occur over the abdomen, buttocks and thighs (see Plate 15). The rash usually begins over abdominal striae. PEP is often very itchy, although topical steroids and antihistamines may partially control this symptom. The condition regresses quickly after delivery.

PRURITUS OF PREGNANCY

This disorder is not associated with a rash, apart from excoriations. It is the result of a cholestasis which normally develops in the last trimester of pregnancy. Affected patients are seldom jaundiced but blood tests will usually show evidence of raised alkaline phosphatase and gamma glutamyl transferase. Pruritus of pregnancy subsides after delivery but tends to recur in subsequent pregnancies. Hydrocortisone cream 1% and systemic antihistamines provide some symtomatic relief.

PEMPHIGOID (HERPES) GESTATIONIS

This is an extremely rare pruritic blistering disorder affecting perhaps 1:40000 pregnancies. Two major factors lead to the development of pemphigoid gestationis. One seems to be a reaction by the mother to the 'non-self', paternally derived, fetal antigens. Secondly the process seems to be subject to hormonal modulation since the use of the oral contraceptive may precipitate relapses.

Papules and urticarial wheals precede the development of blisters; the skin around the umbilicus is frequently affected first. Pemphigoid gestationis can occur at any stage between the second trimester and the puerperium. It frequently recurs in subsequent pregnancies. There are parallels between this disease and bullous pemphigoid. IgG and complement are deposited at the basement membrane zone of the maternal skin. Control of the blistering requires treatment with systemic steroids, although antihistamines and topical steroids may control the pre-bullous stage.

Infections in pregnancy

RUBELLA

Maternal rubella in the first trimester, and particularly the first month, of pregnancy is associated with a high risk of congenital malformation. It is not possible to make the diagnosis with certainty on purely clinical grounds but rubella is characteristically associated with a pink facial macular rash which spreads to involve the trunk and limbs. The rash may be associated with a sore-throat, arthralgia and enlarged occipital lymph-nodes. The diagnosis must be confirmed serologically. If a serum sample is taken when the rash develops and a second sample 7–10 days later should show a fourfold rise in antibody titre. If the patient presents later then the presence of rubella specific IgM in the serum would indicate that primary rubella had occurred in the preceding few weeks.

HERPES SIMPLEX

Babies exposed to primary herpes simplex during delivery should be treated with Acyclovir as should any with clinical evidence of infection. Maternal herpes at the onset of labour is an indication for caesarian section.

Dermatological drugs during pregnancy

It is difficult to state unequivocally that any drug is 'safe' to employ during pregnancy. Table 5.19 shows a list of drugs which are associated with known or probable hazards:

Table 5.19   Known or probable hazards of drugs taken during pregnancy

Etretinate	Teratogenicity
Isotretinoin	Teratogenicity
Tetracyclines	Dental discoloration
Griseofulvin	Foetotoxicity (animals)
Methotrexate	Teratogenicity
Prednisolone (>10 mg)	Fetal adrenal suppression
Dapsone	Neonatal haemolysis
Ketoconazole	Teratogenicity (animals)
Podophyllin	Teratogenicity

Practice points

1 *No surgical or medical treatment will remove stretch marks.*
2 *It is difficult to state unequivocally that any drug is 'safe' to employ during pregnancy.*

Appendices

A1: Treatment and patient advice sheets

Advice for patients with hand eczema

1 While doing dry, dirty work wear cotton gloves to prevent the hands getting excessively soiled.

2 If rubber gloves are worn for wet work remember that sweating inside a glove may be as damaging as the irritation from soap and water. Try not to wear the gloves for more than half an hour at a time. Ideally white cotton gloves should be worn inside loose fitting rubber gloves.

3 Contact between the hands and fruits, vegetables or raw meats can be irritating to the skin and should be minimized. Avoid all contact between inflamed skin and the irritating juices or onions, garlic, citrus fruits and chillies. Once hand eczema is established items that are not normally regarded as damaging, such as potatoes, can provoke further irritation.

4 Do not use household cleansers for cleaning the hands. Avoid contact with organic solvents such as acetone, alcohol and white spirit which can degrease and irritate the skin. When pouring bleaches, acids or detergents be careful that they do not splash onto the hands or forearms.

5 In the home use long handled brushes for dishwashing and for scouring pots, pans and stoves. Nappies and nappy disinfectant can be very irritating; handle soiled nappies with tongs.

6 Avoid prolonged or too frequent washing of the skin. Do not use soaps or cleansers that sting. 'Baby' soaps are usually mild and non-irritating but even the mildest soap must be washed gently and thoroughly off the hands. Remove rings from the fingers when washing the hands. Soap substitutes will probably be prescribed for you and should be used whenever possible.

7 Use the creams and ointments prescribed for you regularly. Renew your supply before it becomes exhausted.

Treatment of scabies

Scabies is an intensely itchy skin disease caused by a small parasite. The condition is quickly and easily cured provided that the treatment is carried out correctly.

1 Apply a thin layer of the insecticide lotion provided with a brush or

sponge. Cover the whole body, except the face and scalp. Do not omit any areas of the skin surface or the treatment may not be successful. Areas such as the finger webs, the middle of the back, and the genitalia are easily forgotten unless care is taken.

2 Leave the medication on for 24 hours and then bath or shower thoroughly.

3 The parasites do not survive away from the skin surface for very long but it is usually recommended that once treatment is completed patients should use fresh under-clothing and bed-linen. This eliminates the very small chance of being reinfected from parasites remaining on clothing. (Normal cleaning or laundering is sufficient; no special disinfection is required).

4 Scabies is transferred from one person to another by close contact. It is therefore important to treat the whole family together *whether they appear to be affected or not.*

5 A single treatment is almost certainly sufficient for a complete cure but you can make absolutely certain by repeating the procedure in one week.

6 The itch of scabies will persist for 10 to 14 days after successful treatment. Do not use the insecticide application more than twice since this is unnecessary and may worsen the irritation.

7 The treatment given to babies and children under 2 years of age is slightly different. It is necessary to treat the scalp and face, whilst carefully avoiding the eyes. The application should be left on for only 8 hours before being washed off. Do not treat babies and children more than once without specific instructions from your doctor.

Remember always treat the whole body and treat the whole family.

Advice for patients with ano-genital pruritus

1 Keep the area clean by washing night and morning. If anal irritation is particularly troublesome then the area should also be washed after each bowel action.

2 Avoid rubbing with a bar of soap or rough flannel. Soap remaining in the skin creases can be very irritating. After washing a thorough rinse with warm water is essential.

3 Keep the area dry. Dab the skin gently with a towel or soft paper. Do not rub. A hairdryer is a gentle way of drying thoroughly.

4 Avoid excessive moisture. Wear cotton underwear not nylon. For women a loose skirt is better than tight jeans. Avoid tights; wear stockings or crotchless tights.

5 Avoid ointments and creams unless specifically prescribed by the doctor. Greasy preparations are undesirable since they may make the skin soggy. Many 'over the counter' products from chemists contain chemicals like local anaesthetics which can cause allergy.

6 The ferocious irritation that develops in this condition almost invariably leads to scratching. Although there may be temporary relief ultimately the condition is aggravated. Avoid scratching if at all possible.

7 If the condition improves it will gradually be possible to reduce the strict regime described above. If the condition returns, as it may do from time to time, start the routine again until the irritation is controlled.

How to undertake contact short dithranol treatment

You will be supplied with:

1 Dithranol in Lassar's paste: 0.25%, 0.5%, 1%, 2%, 3%, 4%, 5%

2 'Dithrocream': 0.1%, 0.25%, 0.5%(Forte), 1%(HP), 2%

Dithranol paste, or cream should only be applied to the areas directed by the nurse or doctor. These will normally be the raised plaques. Apply about 1 mm thickness of the dithranol preparation accurately to the plaques. Do not apply the dithranol to the face, groin, arm-pit or the skin under the breasts. Keep dithranol away from the eyes.

1 Dust each plaque with talc after application to prevent spread of dithranol to uninvolved skin.

2 After 30−60 minutes remove the dithranol. To minimize side-effects like burning make sure that the preparation is thoroughly removed. A cream or ointment can be washed off in a bath or shower. To remove dithranol paste soak a piece of cotton wool in liquid paraffin or corn oil and gently rub the plaques. After the paste is removed wash the areas very well.

Dithranol does tend to stain the skin a reddish-brown colour but this subsides when treatment is stopped. Stains on wall-paper and paint will be more permanent! It is advisable to wear old clothes during treatment because of the staining.

If there is no improvement after 5 days employ a stronger dithranol preparation as advised by the doctor. If soreness or burning develop suspend treatment, apply 1% hydrocortisone cream, and then after 48 hours restart at the last strength dithranol that you could tolerate.

A2: Formulary

The majority of patients with skin disorders will be treated exclusively with proprietary preparations. Only a very limited number of topical treatments mentioned in the text are worth asking the pharmacist to make up.

1 Coal tar pomade

Coal Tar Solution	6%
Salicylic acid	2%
Tween 20	1%
Emulsifying Ointment to	100%

100 g: for use in scalp psoriasis

2 SCC scalp ointment

Precipitated sulphur	1%
Pulverized camphor	2%
Liquid Phenol	2%
Salicylic acid	2%
Emulsifying base to	100%

100 g: for use in scalp psoriasis

3 Betamethasone mouth wash

Betamethasone sodium phosphate	5 g
Chloroform water	50 ml
Mucilage of tragacanth	50 ml

The patients should hold 10 ml in the mouth for 10 minutes and then spit out. Repeat 3 times daily.
100 ml: for use in oral lichen planus

4 Tetracycline mouth wash

The contents of 10 250 mg capsules to be dissolved in 100 ml water. The patient should hold 10 ml in the mouth for 10−15 minutes.

Repeat 3 times daily for 3 days.

100 ml: for use in aphthous and other oral ulcers.

5   Thiabendazole ointment

Triturate two 0.5 g tablets in 10 g white soft paraffin. Apply daily for 5 days.

6   Urea paste 40%

Urea	60.0 g
White bees wax	7.5 g
Wool fat	30.0 g
White soft paraffin	37.5 g
Silica gel H	15.0 g

Protect periungual skin with strapping. Apply paste to nail plate. Cover with Blenderm and further strapping. Leave for 7–10 days.

A3: UK support organizations for patients with skin disorders

ARC, Lupus Booklet, 41 Eagle Street, London W1R 4AR (The Arthritis and Rheumatism Council (ARC) produces a useful handbook for sufferers from SLE)

Albino Fellowship, 15 Goukscroft Park, Ayr KA7 4DS

Coeliac Society, PO Box 220, High Wycombe, Bucks HP11 2HY (Produces a leaflet on dermatitis herpetiformis)

DEBRA (Dystrophic Epidermolysis Bullosa Research Association), 1 King's Road, Crowthorne, Berks RG11 7BG

Disfigurement Guidance Centre (Founder: Doreen Trust), 52 Crossgate, Cupar Fife KY15 5HS

Hairline (Sec Ms E Steel), Hill Vellacott, Post & Mail House, Colmore Circus, Birmingham B4 6AT

National Eczema Society, Tavistock House East, Tavistock Square, London WC1H 9SR

The Neurofibromatosis Association, Surrey House, 34 Eden Street, Kingston upon Thames, Surrey KT1 1ER

Psoriasis Association, 7 Milton Street, Northampton, NN2 7JG

Raynaud's Association Trust, 40 Bladon Crescent, Alsager, Cheshire ST7 2BG

Scleroderma Society, c/o Mrs A.C. Bridgewater, 32 Wensleydale Road, Hampton, Middlesex TW12 2LW

Terence Higgins Trust Ltd, BM, AIDS, London WC1N 3XX

Vitiligo Group, PO Box 919, London SE21 8AW

Bibliography

A large number of excellent dermatology text-books are available. My method of selection has been to list those I use personally for reference.

Baran R. and Dawber R. (Ed). *Diseases of the Nails and their Management.* Blackwell Scientific Publications, Oxford, 1984

Frain-Bell W. (Ed). *Cutaneous Photobiology.* Oxford University Press, Oxford, 1985

Griffiths W.A.D. and Wilkinson D.S. (Ed). *Essentials of Industrial Dermatology.* Blackwell Scientific Publications, Oxford, 1985

Harper J.I. *Handbook of Paediatric Dermatology.* Butterworths, Guildford, 1985

Hughes G.R.V. *Connective Tissue Diseases* (3rd edn). Blackwell Scientific Publications, Oxford, 1987

Rook A. and Dawber R. (Ed). *Diseases of the Hair and Scalp* Blackwell Scientific Publications, Oxford, 1982

Rook A., Wilkinson D.S., Ebling F.J.G., Champion R.H. and Burton J.L. (Ed). *Textbook of Dermatology* (4th edn). Blackwell Scientific Publications, Oxford, 1986

Verbov J. *Essential Paediatric Dermatology* Clinical Press, Bristol 1988

Index